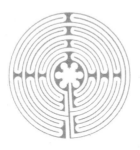

BREAKING THE SPELL OF BINGE-EATING

D1560122

Breaking the Spell of Binge-Eating

A ROAD TO BALANCE IN YOUR LIFE

Joanna Kortink

TRANSLATED FROM THE DUTCH
BY ANITA MILLER

Academy Chicago Publishers

First English Edition
published in 2008 by
Academy Chicago Publishers
363 West Erie Street
Chicago, Illinois 60610

Ninth edition

Published by arrangement with Servire, Kosmos-Z+K Publishers,
Utrecht/Antwerp
© 2006, 2008 Joanna Kortink
Translation © 2008 Anita Miller

Printed and bound in the U.S.A.

All rights reserved.
No part of this book may be reproduced in any form, print or electronic,
without the express written permission of the publisher.

Library of Congress Cataloging-in-Publication Data

Kortink, Joanna.
  [Uit de ban van eetbuien. English.]
  Breaking the spell of binge eating : a road to balance in your life /
Joanna Kortink. — 1st English ed.
      p. cm.
  "Published by arrangement with Servire, Kosmos-Z+K Publishers,
Utrecht/Antwerp."
  Includes bibliographical references.
  ISBN 978-0-89733-577-5 (pbk.)
  1. Compulsive eating. I. Title.
  RC552.C65K6713 2008
  616.85'26—dc22
                        2008037436

*To all my clients, former clients and everybody else
who longs to live life to the fullest!*

Our deepest fear is not that we are inadequate.
Our deepest fear is that we are powerful beyond measure.
It is our light, not our darkness, that most frightens us.
We ask ourselves, who am I to be brilliant, gorgeous,
talented and fabulous?
Actually, who are you not to be?
You are a child of God.
Your playing small doesn't serve the world.
There's nothing enlightened in playing small,
We are all meant to shine, as children do.
We were born to make manifest the glory of God that is
within us.
It is not just in some of us, but it's in everyone.
And as we let our own light shine, we unconsciously give
other people permission to do the same.
As we are liberated from our own fear, our presence
automatically liberates others.

— *Nelson Mandela, inaugural speech 1994*
(based on the poem by Marianne Williamson)

Contents

THE JOURNEY

COMING HOME

Acknowledgements

I have been influenced by many very special people. First of all, I would like to thank my parents, brother and sisters, from whom I received many lessons in living. I want to thank my partner Gerrit, the children and aunt Maria for their support.

Further I want to thank the following: Christa Althof, Gemma Boormans, Martijn van de Graaf, Thea van Liempd, Greta Noordenbos, Ruud Oderkerk, Bibi Stam, Erica and Ruud de Thouars, and Marijke de Waal-Malefijt.

A special thank you to Elise van Riet, who after reading the manuscript together with me extensively went through the whole text and acted as a sounding board.

I would also like to thank Eric Miller and Jordan Miller for believing in my work and for making it possible for me to have my book published.

Many thanks to all of the teachers who have crossed my path, both during my studies, in my dreams and whom I met in every conceivable (and inconceivable) way. Those who I have had the privilege of coaching have also been my teachers. They allowed me to observe them and learn from them and I sincerely hope there will be many years like this in the future.

I am filled with gratitude; this book was in part made possible because of your courage and openness.

Foreword

This book is based on the author's many years of experience with women who suffer from compulsive eating. It is a self-help book that contains various practical exercises and tips to help improve the reader's self-image and her perception of her body. I think these are the most relevant aspects of eating disorders. In the 1997 international bestseller, *The Secret Language of Eating Disorders*, Peggy Claude-Pierre describes the negative and self-destructive thoughts of people who struggle with binge eating: what she calls the inner critic.

Joanna Kortink writes that, earlier, in the 1980s, she herself was conscious of an "inner saboteur" and discovered a way to deal with it. Years later, she was pleased to find her theories confirmed by Peggy Claude-Pierre. Based on her own experiences, Joanna offers in her book, various ways to turn strong negative self-criticism into positive thoughts. Self-acceptance and a positive self-image of the body are the important goals of this book.

The exercises that are described here have a strong connection with cognitive behavioral therapy, now most important in the treatment of people with eating disorders. Methods used in these exercises are also based on recent developments in mindfulness therapy.

This book has a very personal approach and is simply written. It can be used by both professionals (social workers, therapists) and women who suffer from binge eating. Naturally, this book does not claim to be a cure-all for people with serious eating disorders.

Joanna Kortink strongly urges those who suffer from serious eat-ing disorders to seek professional help. However, it is clear from the interviews and examples given here that this book can help to break through negative thought patterns which can strongly influence the lives of women who struggle with binge eating. These women can feel more positive about themselves and their bodies and overcome compulsive eating.

This book is an important self-help book aimed at conquering compulsive eating behavior.

DR. GRETA NOORDENBOS

Dr. Greta Noordenbos of Leiden University is an expert in the field of eating disorders

Introduction

This book is the result of a search within myself and of many years of working with clients who were trapped in self-destructive behavior. In 1987, I started my own practice, in which I helped people with diverse problems, including eating disorders. After ten years, my target group consisted only of people with eating problems who followed what I call "The consciousness training." To explain how this training developed, I will describe how I got there.

I suffered not only from anorexia, but for the longest time from bulimia as well. I know from my own experience how difficult it is to get rid of this. At the end of the seventies, I was sent home after short standard therapy and told that I would have an eating disorder for the rest of my life and I would have to learn to live with it.

To find my own answer, I became a therapist specializing in "the bio-psychosocial aspects of bulimia." I began my own practice and started with workshops. In this way, I could follow my impulses and develop my own way of working.

But after I finished my studies and took several different complementary training courses, I still had the feeling that there was something missing. No matter how deep certain experiences were, they didn't stick. But then I discovered dreams. They showed me the direct way to wholeness. Through my dreams I discovered that I had two me's, each of whom lived in a completely different world. At night I came more and more in contact with my true self, with what fulfilled me deeply, while during the day I lived in a bunker of illusions that consisted of little internal negative voices fighting to get the most attention. Since, in my dreams, I was sometimes a spectator, I taught myself to be a spectator more often during the day. I discovered that it was not life itself, but my way of thinking, that kept me from the fulfillment that I sometimes could feel intensely at night. Through this discovery, I started to feel more free and happier.

What can you expect from this book?

Often I hear: "If only I could get rid of my eating problem, I would be happy." But most people are not unhappy because they have an eating problem, they have an eating problem because they feel unhappy. The eating behavior is usually not an isolated problem, but more often an expression of an underlying problem. That's why it is of major importance to search for the deeper meaning of this problem. People who demonstrate compulsive eating behavior have lost contact with themselves. They can search for a wonder pill or a wonder diet, or they can let themselves be led by instructions, skills and facts, but only after they no longer search for answers outside themselves will their lives be different.

Many factors play a role in the development of compulsive eating behavior. Eating addiction is very complicated, compared to other forms of addiction. We can live without alcohol, cigarettes or TV, but obviously we can't do without food. This means that every day you are confronted with this love/hate relationship. Many books have been written about compulsive eating behavior: ego-documents, manuals for therapists and self-help books. This book belongs to the last category. The most common method used by conventional therapists is cognitive behavioral therapy. Scientific research tells us that approximately half the target group profits from this technique. You will find this form of therapy in most self-help books. I decided to develop a broader approach which I call "The consciousness training." This training is based on the belief that completeness goes further than healthy eating habits: it has a physical, emotional, mental and spiritual aspect.

This book is not a scientific treatise with statistics and tables, but more a travel log. I learn from my clients what really works. I let my clients speak. I give many examples from my practice of the think-and-feel world described by people who demonstrate compulsive eating behavior and the road they took step-by-step to healing. I hope that "Freedom from Compulsive Eating" will be a compass on your inner journey, and, at the same time, I realize that there are many roads which lead to Rome. Feel free to apply whatever appeals to you and leave the rest for what it is. At the same time, I would like to emphasize that I didn't write this book to present a complete description of compulsive eating behavior. How can my understanding about this ever be complete?

There is always more to learn and to understand.

For whom is this book intended?

This book is, in the first place, a resource for people with compulsive eating behavior, but it is also suitable for people who:

- lose and gain weight
- eat for emotional reasons
- associate eating with feelings of guilt
- whose thoughts regularly are dominated by eating or not eating
- are personally involved with somebody who is struggling with eating
- are professionally involved with this problem

The essence of this book is to find yourself again and to live your life according to your true nature. Then you should experience self-confidence, security, strength, wisdom and happiness and be capable of making choices by which you are true to yourself.

Even if you don't have an eating problem, this book can mean a lot to you. Many people experience addiction to alcohol, sex, TV, cigarettes, work, the internet or shopping, don't they? All these forms of addiction have the same pattern. Feeling fat is interchangeable with feeling insecure, unattractive, useless, abandoned and so on. So even if you can't identify with the struggle involving eating, you may identify with the pattern.

I refer to someone with compulsive eating behavior as "she." The reason for this is that by far it is women who struggle with this. Nevertheless, although I write mainly for women, this book is also intended for men with compulsive eating behavior. I learned a lot from the many people whom I was allowed to coach to full recovery from their eating disorder. I consider it a big privilege to have been a witness, time and again, as someone's true personality emerges. One woman described herself as a flower which has opened. With her permission and that of other clients, in this book, I used many examples from my practice and notes from my clients' diaries. To protect their privacy I changed their names. I added some quotations based on notes from sessions and workshops.

How to use this book

- It can be tempting to dip into parts of the book, but the chance for success is greater when you start with the first chapter, because it is important to read the book step-by-step.
- After you have read the first chapter, you will notice its effect in a subtle way.
- Trust that every chapter will give you enough energy to go on.
- You can take this book in like food, just as if you are binging: quickly consuming without really tasting the food. Each chapter consists of four bites.

  Digestion takes time. After each bite, which ends with an exercise, you have to chew a while. If you allow yourself that extra time, you will receive more nourishment from it.

- Many people, especially sensitive individuals, experience a world in almost every word they read. If you notice that you are getting overfed, it can be meaningful to stop reading and go on with it later. Put the book aside for a while to let its contents influence you.
- If you choose to do the exercises at a certain routine time, it becomes a habit. It is also convenient to couple certain exercises to certain moments; that will prevent your forgetting to do them.
- It is possible to ask someone for help, someone you trust and who is sympathetically prepared to think with you and to support you in this process.
- You can be enthusiastic about this book in the beginning, perhaps because you recognize something and experience some support, but as soon as you don't have the feeling that you are being taken seriously, or if you feel challenged, you might be tempted to throw the book aside and to think: "This is another one which is not helping." People with eating problems often think in terms of all or nothing. Don't let that keep you from picking it up again when the time is right.
- Healing starts with self-observation. You will make improvements if you take time every day to go to your inner self. You can do that, for instance, by taking a walk outside in pleasant surroundings; taking a long bath; practice relaxation exercises or writing in a diary.
- Awareness is the first essential step if you want to leave your eating problems behind, but you will reach your goal by not only reading this book, but also by living it.

  You can benefit from this book only if you know the fundamentals well and do the exercises on a regular basis. Repeating the exercises will increase their effectiveness.
- Take sufficient time for an exercise and make sure you can be alone when you do it.

- For some exercises you will need pen and paper, on which you can also write down your insights and changes of attitude.
- Remember, however, that although this is a self-help book, that doesn't mean that there are ready-to-use recipes in it. This is not a cookbook, but a therapeutic guide.
- No book can replace the help of a professional therapist when it comes to healing a serious eating disorder. Use this book as a motivating source to improve your situation and to help you to work with therapists in a effective way. Ask if the therapist wants to read it, too.
- There are four learning stages that are convenient to keep in mind: unaware-incapable, aware-incapable, aware-capable and, at last, unaware-capable. It takes time to learn the fundamentals well, so be patient with yourself.

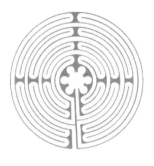

THE WISH TO GO ON A JOURNEY

1

A LOOK AT COMPULSIVE EATING BEHAVIOR

---

*Recognizing that you have an eating problem
is the first step on the road to healing.*

Portrait of a compulsive eater

You are more than your eating problem.

A possible picture of what the life looks like of someone who feels trapped by regularly returning eating binges.

Here is an example from Sandra:

> "I'm at home and I'm feeling good. Suddenly I think of chocolate and before I know it I have eaten all the chocolate in the house. And as if that's not enough, I eat all the cookies too. Or I'm walking down the street, I'm not hungry at all, but suddenly I think about ice cream and feel restless. Where is the nearest ice cream parlor?
>
> Another scenario is that "I go to visit a friend. I'm having a good time. She serves a delicious and healthful meal. I'm full, but as soon as I get home I go to the refrigerator, open it and start eating all kinds of things. Then I begin to call myself names because again I have eaten too much and I think,' I'm too fat. How stupid I must be that I can't control myself.' I know I will never get rid of it. My hand or my thoughts go in the direction of food while I'm not hungry. I'm thinking about eating or about my figure in situations where I shouldn't be having those kinds of thoughts. For instance, I'm talking to somebody and suddenly I lose track of what we were talking about, because

I'm convinced that the other person is thinking that I'm too fat.
Or I'm in a meeting and I can't concentrate any longer because
there is only one thing I'm thinking of: the desire to eat something delicious. If I give in to this I feel guilty the whole time,
and if I don't I have to fight hard against it."

Compulsive eating is more than an activity. It is a predomi-
nant condition of the mind, by which many people are completely
overcome. People with an eating problem can be skinny, fat or in
between. Underlying emotional problems can be diverse and don't
always have to be complicated. Other factors play a role as well. In
this book, I will fully discuss all these matters. Compulsive eating behavior can alternate with periods of severe dieting. Then too,
someone can regularly vomit and/or use laxatives and possibly
exercise excessively. Binge eating, vomiting and the use of laxatives
are done mostly in secret because of shame.

Even the partner, parents or best friends very often know nothing about this behavior. People like Sandra can unexpectedly send
an excuse to avoid a gathering of some sort because they have a
fat-and-ugly attack or because food is their biggest friend at that
moment. Because of this, they find themselves in social isolation.
At the start of the training, my clients often have a problem with
concentrating, which is not surprising if your mind is constantly
preoccupied with food. They think they are too fat, even if that's
not the case. They have an opinion about an "ideal body" and think
that their own body does not meet that standard.

Most people who are in training have, in various ways, denied
themselves food and followed all kinds of diets. They demand a
great deal of themselves: that they can't control their eating behavior, they consider a lack of self-control and will-power. I think differently about this. If you are not hungry and still yearn for food,
most of the time there is a deeper need to which attention should
be paid.

I regularly get questions from new clients about whether I have tips so that they can get started right away. I have included these in the appendix 1. They are also useful when someone is about to have a relapse.

The role that food plays in our lives

There is always a reason to eat.

Reasons to eat

There are different reasons to start eating. First of all, you eat when you are hungry. Apart from that, social events and habits encourage eating. Then, too, food can provide a method to reward, punish or comfort ourselves. To most people, eating is important in life. Food means safety, comfort and love. Normally speaking, breast feeding or bottle feeding can provide physical and emotional rest. Therefore it is not surprising that as an adult we grasp for food when we have a difficult time. In our culture, we are used to the fact that pain is something bad which we have to get rid of quickly. After a spill, a child gets candy and, later in life, many people comfort themselves and others with something delicious when they are feeling miserable. In the same way as alcohol, cigarettes and drugs, food can be used as an escape from unpleasant feelings.

Linda's story

> Linda: "I eat when luck is against me, when I'm feeling insecure, bored, angry, or sad. I devour everything in sight when I don't want to feel unpleasant things from the past. I eat away my loneliness. I fill that void with food. I comfort myself with food

> when things are not going well at work, but also when I'm feel-
> ing euphoric because something is going very well. I eat when I
> experience tension in my relationship with my partner."

Everybody knows at least one way to numb oneself. Many people relate to the habit of using food for different reasons than to
appease physical hunger.

However, eating becomes a problem when it is our way of keeping ourselves on our feet. And that happens when problems, emotions and tensions are being solved with food. Then we gorge ourselves in order to get rid of difficult and unacceptable feelings, like
anger stemming from fear of rejection. It subdues our sorrow, our
loneliness, and the feeling of not being good enough.

Linda told me that in the week between the first meeting and
the first session, she had one spell of binge eating after another. She
thought, "Now it is still allowed, but after the start of the training
it will not be allowed any more." A part of Linda wanted to get rid
of her eating problem as soon as possible, but when she made an
attempt to eat healthy, she could not hold on to that intention for
even a week. Because something else was going on, it was important for that part of her to hold onto binge eating. It is like trying to
go forward with one foot on the accelerator, and the other foot on
the brake. To punish ourselves for this is preposterous. On the contrary, we should pay attention to this reaction in order to understand it. Insight is the first step to different behavior. I told Linda I
appreciated her openness and asked her if there were more factors
that led to binge eating.

Habits:

> "When I'm watching television or when I'm reading, there has
> to be something to nibble on. The weekend starts on Friday
> night and that is the start of the eat feast. Mostly, I dread study-
> ing. To postpone that a little while, I usually eat something

first. Automatically, as soon as I'm tired, I eat sweets. While I'm waiting for the train I buy sweets. It was an eye-opener when I found out how many times I eat something out of habit. Many activities are automatically coupled to food and I don't notice when I put it in my mouth."

Messages she received as a child about eating:

"I always had to clean my plate, then I was a good girl. When I was left alone I got a treat. When I was naughty I got punished by not getting candy that day. Something delicious was always eaten in one sitting (licorices, a box of chocolate, a package of cookies, ice cream). I was comforted by a piece of pie if something nice suddenly did not happen.

In the past, there was always something sweet when my parents left me alone. I realize that as soon as I'm alone I still have the tendency to put something sweet in my mouth."

Also, she had repeating thought patterns:

"Calorie-rich food is bad and forbidden. Healthy and moderate eating is equivalent to being on a diet. If someone offers me something to eat I say "yes" because I don't want to hurt the person's feelings. Without something sweet it is not cozy. I eat too much for fear of being hungry. There are various thoughts about eating which stand in my way. Because that brings on a lot of stress . . . I start to eat again and that frustrates me."

These examples show that there are a lot of reasons for compulsive eating. It takes time to change an ingrained habit.

After all, it took years before eating became a problem. Solving it requires patience, love and wisdom. The challenge here is not to set the task to oneself too high.

It is important to take small, realizable steps. To eat differently is a learning process that is like falling down and standing up again.

Failures don't exist, there are only experiences which give us a chance to look at the problem differently the next time.

Exercise: two scripts

Write two scripts about what your life could be like five years from now. Write in the present tense. Include themes such as food, body, family, finances, health, relaxation, partner, classes, friendships, and living arrangements. Write one script in which you describe what your life will be like if you do nothing to get better and become more and more caught in a vicious circle. The other script describes your new life in which you are completely healed! It should describe what your life will look like when it expresses your innermost hopes and dreams. You could write these scripts in the form of a letter to a friend (imaginary or real). An example by Claudine:

Fragments from the negative script:

. . . One day in this life is more than I can handle. Even the tiniest efforts are too much for me. Basically, walking is too tiring . . . I often have stomach aches, my esophagus is sore, I regularly have headaches. . . .

Mentally, I feel dead and cold. Television, sounds, too many people are all noise to me. I can't stand it. The only things I am able to enjoy are my secret eating binges, but then only for a short while . . . I have a terrible self-image. I am a fat, gluttonous pig, I have no self-control. I just wear any old thing (practically nothing fits anymore) as long as it's big. I avoid looking at myself. I'm disgusted by myself, hate myself . . . I have no plans for the future. My thoughts are clouded by a thick, heavy, cool fog. I can't concentrate on my classes, my thoughts are sluggish, I am too tired. All the nice things in life are over-shadowed by exhaustion, numbness, feelings of guilt and shame. Basically, I am totally burnt out; I might as well lie down and die. I just vegetate. . . .

Fragments from the positive script:

"I have a lot of energy, no pain . . . I have a figure that suits me, I eat consciously and healthy and enjoy it. Mentally I'm stable . . . I'm happy with my good and less good qualities. I can now laugh at myself when I unintentionally say or do something. I have left behind pain from the past. I save my energy for matters I really think are important . . . Every day I do relaxation exercises. Because of that I'm empty and fresh. Our sexual and intimate relationship is harmonic. I dare to trust myself and discover new things on a regular basis. In contact with others, I watch my boundaries . . . I accept my parents' peculiarities . . . I have inspiring friends with whom I can be myself . . . I have many interests . . . Sorrow and set-backs will always be there, but I can cope with them. I love myself, I deserve to have a nice life."

The cause of compulsive eating behavior

The shortest road to suffering is to avoid suffering.

Inner emptiness

People always ask me: "What is the cause of my eating problem?" It is a myth to think that the cause is the desire to be slender, anything one's parents may have done, sexual abuse or any other trauma. Each one of these can play a role in an eating disorder, but the real cause lies much deeper. Just as fever and a rash are symptoms of the measles, so is compulsive eating behavior a symptom of a deeper lying cause. It is my opinion that people who suffer from binge eating have lost themselves and are living with an unreal self-image.

There are many strategies people use to avoid the inner emptiness caused by this unreal self-image: one is compulsive eating behavior. Later, I will deal with factors that play a role in compulsive eating behavior; here, however, I will limit myself to inner emptiness and predisposition.

From the first day of our lives we are completely dependent on love, attention and care from other people. Due to this dependency, we inevitably meet frustration and pain, because our needs and longings are not always fulfilled. Even if we grow up in a loving environment, we will experience frustrations. Sometimes we do not receive the desired attention as quickly as we want it. A classic example is the baby who cries because he wants to be fed. If a child cries a couple of times and it does not get what it wants, it finally gives in. If its needs are not sufficiently satisfied, a feeling of inner emptiness develops.

Instead of accepting the fact that suffering is part of life, in our urge to survive we do everything to avoid less pleasant experiences. In that way we unconsciously develop a survival strategy.

Overeating can be a method of keeping our feet on the ground. Other ways are seeking escape in alcohol, in overwork, or spending hours watching TV. Everybody knows strategies that can be used to avoid the feeling of inner emptiness that began in childhood. This can be compared to pain from a deep wound that we try to relieve with a narcotic. But when the medication is no longer effective, we feel the pain again, because the wound is still there. The pain goes on as long as we don't take care of the wound.

Not only do we usually feel inadequate, but it can add to our frustration when we "drop the ball." People disappoint us and we behave disappointingly ourselves; nobody is perfect. Others don't always listen to us attentively, but we are not always good listeners either. We are being rejected and we feel that rejection. Without realizing it, we can behave like a "wounded child." That child is in every one of us and it pops up to the surface at the most inconvenient moments. Deep inside us we can feel hurt, lonely, helpless and dependent.

This can express itself in different ways: as in eating problems, addictive behavior, problematic relationships, depression, physical complaints and loss of energy.

Besides all this, our circumstances in life are not always what we should like them to be. We will find ourselves again when we no longer chase perfection, but accept reality about ourselves and the world. There is a difference between who we are and who we want to be. By changing irrational thoughts into realistic ones and by abolishing emotional blocks, the fog that developed in the past will be erased and we will view our lives from a different perspective.

Born with a certain predisposition

The reason why one develops compulsive eating behavior as a survival strategy is connected with the environment in which we have grown up and with our personal predisposition. We are all born with a certain predisposition. The structure is present in the embryo and expresses itself physically in the form of a certain stature and biological vulnerability, and mentally in the form of specific characteristics. Examples of characteristics that I observe in compulsive eating behavior are perfectionism, lack of self-esteem, impulsiveness and insecurity. The experience of my therapeutic work teaches me that many clients are very sensitive.[1] Everyone is sensitive, some more than others, but one in five are highly sensitive. With their delicate character, these people have a special antenna that registers subtle signals from their environment.

With this predisposition, which is a gift, they can detect more than others, feel when something is not right, notice more quickly what the environment needs. Because they are attuned to receiving subtle signals, their organism is more quickly affected by crude stimuli. Think of noise, bright lights, too much activity, crude treatments or negative moods. Because of their specific predisposition, these people are more likely to react to certain foods in a negative way (especially when sugar or artificial ingredients are added). They can also be very sensitive to medicines. They can then be quickly overwhelmed and need time to rest and recover. Hypersensitivity is not always recognized as such, even though this can make people more susceptible to developing an eating problem.[2]

Choosing the light or the darkness

Janine: "I saw my future as one big void. It became clear to me that I could choose light or darkness. For the first time I had the feeling that I was no longer out of control, but capable of steering my own course. I saw myself standing at a crossroads where I could decide which direction to choose. It was suggested to me that at night before going to sleep I should call up my picture of what I wanted my life to look like. That way there came light in the darkness and I felt confidence in my future."

Many people think: As soon as I get rid of my eating problem, I will be happy. But most people are not unhappy because they have an eating problem, they have an eating problem because they are unhappy. As soon as we no longer look at the eating problem as an isolated problem, but look at it from a larger perspective, then we make way for healing. Especially when we emphasize the disturbed eating behavior and work hard on that, we confirm our inability. That doesn't do us any good. If, however, we are prepared to acknowledge our unlimited abilities, our strength breaks free. Although it is important to look at the future full of trust, it is not realistic to be completely focused on the future, because then we will never be happy.

Janine showed that the present offered far more possibilities than she could ever have imagined. After doing a "positive script" writing exercise, I encouraged her to translate this into a collage. Every night as she lay in bed, Janine looked at her collage and imagined what she would like to be like. She told me that her eldest sister was going to throw a big party and that she wanted to feel at this party the way she planned to feel in the future. She wanted to experiment with this thought and decided to behave that night as if she was already the way she wanted to be.

The next session a radiant Janine walked in. She had enjoyed an unforgettable party.

In the past she had behaved like someone who basically wanted to make herself invisible, but now she dared to go up to and chat with many guests. She felt free, energetic and enjoyed the party immensely. Where before she had kept quiet when she was eating with others (out of fear that someone would say she was too fat), she dared at that moment to talk and then to eat a little and to enjoy it. Once at home she didn't start eating, something she had done habitually after a dinner party, but now she felt deeply fulfilled.

Exercise: to see your ideal life before your eyes.

Making a collage is an aid to forming the picture of your future.

Collect pictures and prints of images that show how you would like your life to look. Make a collage of those, and look at it every night. You can draw little balloons coming from your mouth which contain short, positive statements just like in a comic book.

Look at this collage before going to sleep. Continue with closing your eyes and picture which positive thoughts you have, what you shall see and feel when all this becomes reality.

Proceeding from overeating to living in full

Finding yourself again is to see your life
from another perspective.

The inward journey: searching for who you really are

Seeking to discover why you are so desperately longing for food can be the beginning of a deep healing process, a voyage of discovery into yourself in which you are going to search for who you really are. Central to this book is this "inner voyage." You can compare this transformation process to a labyrinth (look at the image on the cover of this book) which is a symbol for the path of life. It helps you to get to know yourself. This labyrinth consists of only one path that finds the way to itself, leads to the centre and then makes its turns to the exit. Unlike a maze, there are no paths with a dead end. In a maze we direct our attention outward to find the way, while in a labyrinth it is the inner experience that is important. The clients who took this voyage learned to listen to their real thoughts, feelings and longings. During their journey along this turning and winding path, there were moments when they felt happy, relaxed, satisfied and energetic, but there were also moments when they felt frustrated, lonely, rebellious, sad and lost. But they kept going on, step by step. During this voyage of discovery, they found themselves again. In the centre, where a human being is alone with herself, they found their true character, the essence of who they really are. Here they felt born again and free, but that didn't seem to be the end of the journey. After that, they had to leave the labyrinth to integrate their new perception of being into their everyday life. The Hopi Indians know this labyrinth as a symbol of Mother Earth and death and rebirth. Death is the end of the former way of being; a human being is born again. The voyage of discovery inward goes through a couple of phases:

0. You are feeling unhappy and you wish to do something about it (That is the topic of the next two chapters).

1. The journey through the unknown labyrinth (chapters 3–6).

2. You have accepted your circumstances in life and you feel an inner rebirth.

3. You are leaving the labyrinth and look at your life from a new perspective and in a new light. With full confidence you move towards the future. (Chapter 7 contains the last two phases.)

Below is an explanation of the phases, followed by an example of a client's reaction and a dream fragment. To get to know ourselves very well we need a broader perspective. Dreams can be helpful for this purpose and can be used as a road to healing. They come from the subconscious and can show where the traveler can be found. This produces a supplementary, non-analytical look at the whole thing.

Phase 0

Myra: "I have a demanding job, a relationship and a very extensive circle of friends. I have been suffering from bulimia for 15 years. Recently I got married. During my honeymoon, everything went well as far as eating was concerned, meaning I didn't throw up, because beforehand I had honestly planned not to do that. But now I'm home again and it seems as though nothing has changed. My husband and I would like to have a baby but as a doctor I know that it is better to have healthy eating habits first. I wonder if the problem will go away by itself after I have a baby."

Typical for this phase is that you're feeling unhappy.

At first, compulsive eating seemed like a way to handle daily problems, but now you realize that it is a self-created prison. You are cut off from nourishing sources of life and unapproachable to others. Life is one big punishment, in which everything seems to repeat itself. There is no space for anything new.

Trudy: "In my dream I would love to go on a journey. I have packed everything and I'm on my way. Once at the border, I'm held up by a customs officer who asks to see my passport. Then it seems to my astonishment that I can't prove my legality, because I completely forgot to bring this important document with me. Disappointed, I'm on my way home again."

When you are "in the departure hall" there is always something or someone holding you back when you want to start "the big journey." With Trudy this seemed to be a recurrent theme. The dreams in which she wanted each time to go on a journey and was held back became more and more upsetting. When she had the courage to start on her inner journey this dream theme disappeared.

The first phase

Kate: "I was alone for years and was in a relationship with a married man. I saw him a couple of times a month. For him I wanted to be beautiful and slim. The days before he came I hardly ate anything, to be super slim. But as soon as he was gone, I ate the whole day. Although it was very difficult, I broke up the relationship, because I want a man who will stay with me. I understand that my eating problem is going to interfere with any new relationship, that's why I'm now seriously prepared to do something about it."

Now you decide to act. You are choosing the unknown. You are going on a search for yourself and you are going to find help with this. Not everybody is going to understand what you are doing, but you can find understanding from those who have made such an inner journey themselves. With the leap into the deep, into the unknown, the lonely journey has started.

Cynthia: "I dream that in the middle of the night men with knives have broken into my parents' home. I'm alone and I see them coming towards me. While they try to decide the best strategy to attack me, in this unguarded moment I manage to escape. I'm outside in my bare feet and without a warm coat. I wander through the darkness, I'm cold, but relieved, because precisely at the right moment I made my escape."

With each new phase we have to deal with something or someone who is trying to interfere with us. They always reflect our defenses, our fears and our desires.

The second phase

Eline: "I have one brother, no sisters. I fantasize all the time that I have a sister with whom I would be on the same wavelength, because my brother and I are like oil and water. He was the constant know-it-all and I always went along with him. He kept nagging about my appearance, which made me feel very insecure. Now I see that he is insecure himself and that he tried to hide that by criticizing me. But he finds fault with me less and less, because I don't react anymore."

After a long journey you leave the dark area behind you. You're looking at the past through different eyes. You don't look back in anger anymore, but through insight you accept life as it is. You have reconciled yourself to your destiny. You have found out who you really are and because of that you accept yourself with love and find peace.

> Patty: "I go with my mother to an art exhibit. I recognize the building from a distance, because there is an impressive angel hanging above the entrance. We go in and walk directly to the second floor, because we know that the most beautiful statues and paintings are there. We both enjoy these works immensely. I feel rewarded that I can share this moment with my mother and feel a deep rapport."

Patty had this dream right after she reconciled with her mother.

The third phase

> Valerie: "After my divorce I realized that my happiness no longer depended on having a partner. I'm capable now of enjoying the big and small things in life. Although the longing for a partner still exists, it doesn't feel like a painful loss any more. I know I'm capable of enjoying life on my own."

Now when you see yourself through new eyes, you are capable of distancing yourself from things that don't belong to you anymore and you can open yourself to the here and now.

> Patricia: "I'm wearing a beautiful shining long silk dress, because I'm getting married. Just before entering the church my mother hands me a small wedding bouquet. Many friends and family members came over especially for me. For me alone, because I'm marrying . . . myself!"

This dream fragment reflects the oneness in yourself. This was a brief travel description. I'm not making it prettier than it is; the inner journey requires courage and patience. Sometimes I ask clients during an evaluation to look at the labyrinth that hangs on the wall in the office and to point to where they are right now. Thus, they can see that they have already covered many miles and they can see where they will end if they keep following their path.

The trusted, but limited situation in life

Before we start on the journey through the labyrinth, I invite you to have a look at the "departure hall." The examples show how we can lock ourselves in life as though it were a prison. And the days repeat themselves over and over.

> Elsie: "When I'm feeling miserable, I start to eat, but I eat even when I'm feeling happy. I grow fatter and feel very frustrated by this. I don't want to be like my mother, who now weighs over 200 pounds. I want to lose weight, but the temptation to eat is stronger still. Buying clothes is very frustrating for me, I do it as seldom as possible. The last time that I went shopping and could not find anything, I walked straight to the first baker's shop and bought chocolate and pastry."

> Margaret: "What meaning in life is left for me when I can't eat and drink? I feel down, although I take anti-depressants."

> Bridget: "I have a recurring nightmare in which a tiger is trying to attack me. The tiger becomes more and more aggressive."

> Sylvia: "For many years I have suffered from bulimia. I'm so ashamed of this that I do not dare tell anyone. A little voice in my head says that if I do tell somebody, I will have to do something about it. That's what I'm afraid of, because you hear such negative stories about fighting against it. If I hear or read something about that, I think: it can always be worse."

But the outer world can also be "pleasant." There is always some-one who means well, but who will try to keep you from setting out on your "inner journey."

> Mother talking to daughter: "That digging into yourself brings nothing but misery. You are not going to look for trouble like that, are you?' (And my mother promptly lights another ciga-rette and has a second glass of wine)."

> General practitioner: "You have an eating problem? That's ridiculous. The only thing you have to do is to eat a little less, and then your problem will be solved."

> Girlfriend: "You look good, don't you? What are you worrying about? Oh, well, listen to this: that boy I met recently . . ."

> Partner: "You've already tried so many times. You can't do it. You have to accept the fact that for the rest of your life you will have a problem with this."

Time and time again we can try to escape from our fear, but that will only make it grow more intense. It is better to concentrate on the deep longing for peace and freedom. The first step on the road to healing starts with the recognition that you have an eating problem.

Exercise: letter to the eating problem

Write a friendly letter to the compulsive eater in yourself. Do not write like an enemy. This will help you to gain more insight into the role that compulsive eating plays in your life. To give you an idea of what such a letter could look like, here is a friendly one written by Tessa, followed by a hostile one by her.

Dear Eating Problem,

Thank you for being with me so often. I appreciate
your helping me with all my problems. When I'm feeling
lonely, or tense, you are always there. Because of you I
forget all my difficulties. I don't have to think about anything at all if you are there and all my problems vanish
into thin air. I can always count on you, you never leave
me. From early in the morning until late in the evening
and even at night you are there for me. I never have to
wait for you; as soon as there is a problem, there you are.
I think that's really special. I wouldn't know what to do
without you. You are a great friend.

Love, Tessa

Eating problem,

I hate you. No matter what I do . . . or want to do, I
meet you. You dominate my whole life. Because of you
I'm not myself and I lose control. I loathe my body and
think that others loathe it too. Because of you I have
become very quiet. All day I think of food and calories; getting up with food and going to bed with food.
It drives me crazy. There are constant fights going on in
my head, so I feel very stressed. I don't want that binge
eating anymore. I want to enjoy life again. You obstruct
me much too much, so I don't want to deal with you anymore. Leave me alone. Don't try to persuade me, because
I have made up my mind.

Tessa

2

EATING DIFFERENTLY STARTS WITH THINKING DIFFERENTLY

Most ot the time it's our thought that makes us long for food.

We are hardly ever ourselves; usually we play a role

We have two "Selves": a limited "Self" where we suffer and a true "Self" that stands above this drama.

Introduction

For many people, it is true that as children and later in life we would give anything to be accepted and loved. But when we develop this side of our personality, there can quickly come into existence an opposite pole that rebels against it. That " true" side raises the fear that we will not be accepted with this personality, so many people suppress that desire for acceptance in themselves. They are hardly ever their true selves; they play a role. But what subconsciously they try to suppress doesn't disappear. All those parts, also called partial-personalities, keep their power over us until they are recognized and accepted. When, for instance, you constantly scold "the inner critic" with: "You are not allowed to have candy, because then you will never get a better figure," it is possible that suddenly the "thrill-seeker" in you becomes dominant and indulges itself in food. When we choose one side, sooner or later the other side rebels against it.

This can be compared to a ball that we try with all our might to push under water; with the same power it always pops up to the surface again. If we no longer want to be a plaything of our partial personalities and experience a constant loss, than there is a third possibility. Everyone occasionally examines his own feelings or thoughts. That is the objective observer who has a view from an elevated observation point. From this contemplative position, this non-judgmental witness is aware of the existence of all partial personalities. There is neither repression nor identification. Inherently, these partial personalities possess positive characteristics. However, through disappointment, frustration and pain they can become warped. In this way, a characteristic like conscientiousness can easily turn into perfectionism, and sensitivity can lead to self-effacement. The observer can be a guide to the road back to restoring our characteristics to their original state.

The limited Self

> Helena: "I was criticizing myself once more when Joanna asked which part of me was talking. Again I identified myself with the perfectionist. I can now laugh heartily about it."

Thinking is an internal dialogue with ourselves. It is perfectly normal that thoughts seem like voices in our head which try to explain something from different points of view. Even when we are young children we use fixed thought patterns and "listen" to our own thoughts. As I have said, a problem arises when two partial personalities are in conflict with each other. That conflict can seem to be a real war in our minds. The stress that causes this can be a reason for binge eating, but what is being suppressed doesn't disappear. All these parts continue to exist and to control us. You can compare them to parasites which gradually nestle into your body and aggressively start to suck the life out of you. They are always looking to see when they can attack, and they are especially successful when we feel threatened. But although these partial-personalities are a part of ourselves, they are not our complete selves. Your big toe is a part of you, but you are not that big toe.

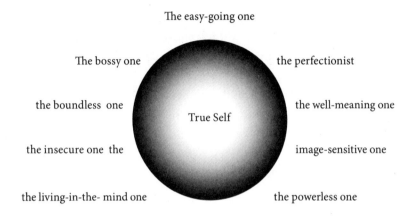

The easy-going one

The bossy one

the perfectionist

the boundless one

True Self

the well-meaning one

the insecure one the

image-sensitive one

the living-in-the- mind one

the powerless one

If we can identify these partial personalities, then we can prevent them from continuing to poison our lives. All these negative inner voices keep us in prison. I call this the "limited-self." I have mapped out nine of the partial personalities as follows.[3]

Here Helen gives examples of each internal little voice.

The perfectionist:

> "Do you really think that one little candy doesn't matter? Do you really think that you can get the ideal body if you can't even realize that you must say no to that candy? It is all or nothing and I'm going for all. So no more sweets, but a lot of fiber. And exercise, not that sloppy twice-a-week workout, but every day. If you are not really doing it well, it will get you nowhere."

This part is really brilliant in delivering a bad feeling to us, because it is always ready to point at what is not perfect. This critic will never forget one detail.

The well-meaning one:

> "If you will only listen to me, you will get there. Just don't eat during the day, only eat in the evening for several weeks, and you'll see how quickly you lose the pounds."

This part seems to be a rescuer in need, but it only helps you get from the shore into the water. It offers short-term solutions, and so failure is inevitable.

The image-sensitive one:

> "What will the world think if they see me like this? If I really want people to admire me, I will have to change a couple of things. With this body I will never get there. First I'm going to town to look for a new slenderizing outfit. That will make me feel better. (Just for a short while, because then there comes 'the poor me')."

The image-sensitive one is living for the external world. Externals are important. It is dependent on admiration by others. That's important for its self-esteem.

The powerless one:

> "I can't help it if my body tells me it needs sweets. Who am I to say no? The craving for food is stronger than I am. Then it is better for me to eat instead of being angry and sad. I can't control it. I want to change, but I won't be successful. I don't know what it is."

This is the "poor-me" part, the ongoing victim. It hopes to be saved, but it is frustrated every time.[4]

The living-in-the-mind one:

> "I'm sitting here safe and sound in my mind. That's how I can oversee and consider everything. I like to put everything in small familiar boxes. That's how I can know what to expect. That way the world is clearly understandable and safe."

This part doesn't like to have disagreeable feelings, so the head has become a haven of refuge.

The insecure one:

> "I'm afraid, afraid to change. I don't know what is going to happen when I do things differently. Who knows what I will have to deal with. What will be the result? I don't know if I dare to change and if I can.

This aspect is the scared one, the suspicious one in all of us. It doesn't have confidence in other people. If there is a chance to act, it will start from the worst scenario.

The boundless one:

> "I want a cookie. No, I want two. Now I have already eaten two, so number three goes as well. One more to unlearn the habit. Well, now it doesn't matter anymore, I might as well eat the whole package. And I'm going to eat that little left-over pudding too. What do I care . . . tomorrow is another day."

It is the boundless one, the pleasure-seeker in us for whom it is never enough. This part runs away from pain. It thinks that rules are annoying and unimportant.

The bossy one:

> "Do you really think that you can succeed? You are fat, clumsy and incapable of finishing anything. In the future you're only going to become fatter and more miserable. Stop, because you'll never get there. You'll never achieve your goal."

This part symbolizes the negative, the nag, the aggressive, the vindictive in us. Vulnerable feelings are suppressed.

The easy-going one:

> "I think it is okay as it is. Why change? The world doesn't stop turning. I don't see any benefit in changing anything at all, I've been doing this for years."

From sheer force of habit this part wants to keep everything as it is, choosing false security instead of taking risks.

Recognizable? These familiar little voices show how we move from one position to the other in this vicious circle. The contradictory voices of our partial personalities maintain the eating problem. What was once a way to protect ourselves, has become a self-created prison. By recognizing the "limited me" in ourselves, the possibility exists that we will no longer be kept in prison by our partial personalities.

The true self

> Wendy: "Like a caterpillar I have formed a cocoon around me and I'm still imprisoned by it. My cocoon-complex forces me to choose that false gray security. Again and again. That exaggerated caution keeps me completely motionless. It keeps me from approaching life with an open mind."

At the start of our awakening process we can be compared to a grub in a cocoon, where life is monotonous and dark. A grub is born with the capability within itself to shed the caterpillar phase and eventually to become a butterfly.

If we are being transformed, just as a butterfly is transformed, then we are in contact with our true self. Then we are living from the heart and intuitively we know what to do and what not to do. Our true self is located in a place where the limited self has no influence. Finding our true self again is a journey from one conscious level to another. It is not something you do or you don't do. Having insight is the key that opens the door here. It asks you to look out of your cocoon to a bigger reality. By consciousness-expanding we can feel just like that butterfly, lively and free, and our existence takes on color. Though many people cling to the caterpillar; they can't imagine what it is like to be transformed into a butterfly.

Wendy is still a prisoner in her cocoon. As a child, she had not yet developed the capacity to see things in the right perspective, and she still believes that she has a limited scope. Many people think and act like that. But we can decide to step out of this vicious circle of functioning unconsciously. This means that to observe, to be really prepared to see what is there—that should be our second nature during this inner journey. A lot of patience is needed for this, because old habits are not easy to overcome.

I, too, felt like a prisoner for years because eating and insecurity about my looks played a predominate role in my life. In spite of receiving many compliments from others, I saw myself completely differently. A turning point in my life was a dream I had in which to my great surprise, I discovered a photo of myself as a radiant woman. This dream showed me that what I thought about myself was wrong. Suddenly I looked at myself with different eyes. I could not deny it, this was me and nobody else. The dream showed me who I really am. This woke me and told me more than anyone or anything had told me before.

Pictures, whether they are from a dream or from being evoked in our mind, can be a source of inspiration, energy and wisdom. In this way, we can train the human mind to come into contact with its true self. To imagine something is a powerful way to make a change, because the subconscious reacts very strongly to this. If I ask my clients in the beginning of therapy to picture themselves as they are at that moment, most of them can do that.

But they are not particularly happy with this image. After that, I invite them to contact their true self, their blueprint. Almost every time a picture appears that radiates openness, light, vitality and tenderness. We can choose on a regular basis to make conscious contact with our natural, radiant being. What you could do, as a reader, is, for example, to find a picture in which you look radiant (even as a child) and look regularly at that picture. Also, you can make a drawing of your true self. In this way you can remind yourself, over and over, who you really are and you can embody this picture. If someone says: "I can't picture myself as radiant," then this person is excluding the possibility that this picture is ever going to become reality.

If, on the contrary, you imagine regularly what you want, then that is a strong support for the realization of this desire.

Babette wrote: "The survey of the partial-personalities was an eye-opener to me. Suddenly, everything came together. For years I have identified myself with traits of character like extreme insecurity and dependency. By choosing during the session to step out of this vicious circle, suddenly 'my true self' appeared: a warm, loving, radiant me whom I recognized from long ago."

Maybe you think I am fooling myself if I suddenly develop that radiant personality with all these beautiful qualities that go with it.

But, working with this, we become sharply aware of how we don't radiate when we hurt ourselves with all those negative thoughts about ourselves and the world. That is just an illusory picture, because it is based on the painful experiences from the past. In that way, many people fool themselves, because the picture they make of themselves is not in keeping with reality.

Limited thoughts, feelings and behavior prevent us from radiating, but when we remove the layer of dust, bit by bit, our real qualities emerge and who we really are becomes visible. This does not mean that you have to be another person to live life to the fullest; what is important is that you shake off your excess baggage. We have a free, radiant character that is undamaged, present behind the cloud cover of all those negative little voices in us. The variety of negative thoughts is as if the clouds have covered the sun, but still the sun shines in all its glory.

> Ricky wrote: "I thought that restlessness was something that was a part of me, until Joanna said: 'This is not who you really are. You are not the person you became, but you are who you really are deep inside yourself.'"

If you are in contact with your true self, then you feel complete, fulfilled and satisfied.

Clarissa Pinkola Estés writes in her book *Women Who Run With the Wolves* about knowing that nature is there for all who are lost. No matter how many times she is suppressed, she always pops up again. We no longer have to be the plaything of external circumstances when we find out who we really are. Then we need no longer depend on others for our inner happiness. Although the circumstances change, the silent witness in ourselves is the timeless, constant factor in the midst of all time-bound changes.

Exercise: who am I for real?

Choose a quiet space in the house that is big enough to hold two imaginary circles, in between which you can walk back and forth. The outmost circle represents your limited self and the inner circle your true self. In the outmost circle you put down pen and paper. You can mark the inner circle, for instance, by placing a chair or cushion in it.

1. Stand in the outmost circle and make contact with the thoughts and emotions from one of the nine partial-personalities whom you know well. Imagine that you exist only as this one little voice. Write down what it tells you. Then do this with the other little voices that you recognize. Learn what the different parts do with you.

2. Now, slowly walk to the inner circle, which represents your true self. Sit down, relax and close your eyes. Soon you will notice that something has changed. This spot is connected with silence and your original qualities. This wise and sincere part is aware of all those partial personalities. Here you can see that you are not the powerless one or the easy-going one. The witness in you does not push them away, but accepts them as they are. They are no more than self-created figments of imagination. Feel the liberation that comes from this.

3. Open your eyes again, and step out of the inner circle. Make contact again with your limited self in the outmost circle. How do you feel about this now? Probably the experience is different now than it was in the beginning. If you feel critical, realize that you are dealing with your inner critic. The more times you practice this exercise on the same spot, the easier it becomes to look closely at the limited self without criticizing it.

Dialogue with the inner saboteur

The influence of the inner saboteur does not decrease when you are running away from it.

How a partial personality can be our boss

The limited self expresses itself in various partial personalities. Sometimes a part, like the perfectionist or the bossy one, can manifest itself, as if it alone is in charge day and night. Such a saboteur has a devastating effect. This one can even try, with hateful remarks, to bring us to the point where we are incapable of seeking help. It can say, "You are already lost, you are not worth helping, nobody cares about your problems. Stupid, fat pig."

Women can "eat away" those nasty thoughts, or they can starve themselves for days in a row until they can't hold out anymore. As a result, many are caught in a vicious circle and start to hate themselves more and more. They try to hide this from the outer world, because they are ashamed of their behavior and don't understand it. That's why they become more and more estranged from themselves. The saboteur came into existence through a survival strategy. It had a function and maybe it still has. Its influence will decrease if one does not run away from it. With me, the reversal originated when I realized years ago that there are no worse enemies than the ones that have nestled themselves in your heart.

At a certain point I grew so tired of this that I spoke out loud against those little negative voices. If the self critic said "Why are you so fat?" I asked myself what my reasonable mind would say and gave a short response. By observing the difference between my limited self and my true self, I gained more and more control over my life. That's how I found the original voice of my heart, the voice that brought me back to myself. To my pleasant surprise, I found out later that a colleague on the other side of the world, Peggy Claude-Pierre, author of the book *The Secret Language of Eating Disorders*, had successfully used the same strategy with her clients.

Being in control

I asked Kathinka, a teacher, if there was ever a pig-headed child in her classroom. She knew precisely what I was implying. She immediately put a stop to that person, because otherwise the classroom would become a big mess. I asked her how she did that.

It came to this: she stood on her authority. She let the person know that she was in charge and not the other. I invited Kathinka to attack her inner saboteur with the same strength that she uses in the classroom. I asked her to stand on a certain spot in the room and to imagine that at that moment she put herself into the place of the rebellious child within herself. She did well, because that voice was familiar to her for years. After she made room for that voice, she placed herself opposite the spot where the inner saboteur had uttered the words. She was thinking of the example of the pig-headed child in her classroom and she was able to look at it very clearly from a distance. She took charge not as "the bossy one" (partial personality) who wanted to control the chaos in the classroom, but in a caring way through authentic strength. Very soon her inner saboteur had nothing to say any longer. Most clients feel controlled for years by such an inner saboteur.

Although all those irrational thoughts are dominant, our true self, which represents the original consciousness, is also there. I ask clients to write down what that inner saboteur tells them and to try to give a "healthy" answer. In that way they can recognize clearly irrational thoughts, find their own strength and distance themselves from the inner saboteur which will thus lose more and more territory. Here are two examples given by Sarah.

INNER SABOTEUR	RATIONAL THINKER
Watching TV. What shall I take upstairs? An apple, and cottage cheese with strawberries, the tea to wash it down and of course cookies and chocolate. Maybe some more crackers, but I'll get them during the commercials. And let's not forget the wine-gums, because I can't live without something to suck on.	I don't have to take anything upstairs because I just have HAD ENOUGH. Shut your mouth, I'M NOT listening to you.

A week later the saboteur feels pressed too hard and starts to attack her.

INNER SABOTEUR	RATIONAL THINKER
You are a good-for-nothing. Everybody is fed up with you. You will never make it. You don't know what you want. You don't know what you think. You don't know what you feel. You are going down the drain. You are always busy with beautiful plans and it brings in nothing. It is only going to be more difficult to get out of it. You are just a heap of misery.	This process takes time and I allow myself that time. I don't have to do a thing and I'm allowed a lot. I will fall on my face many times, but I think you don't have to make things worse than they are. I do the things day by day as I need.

Actually, without personal help, most people can apply this technique. A couple of years ago I presented this technique on paper to Marlies. A week later, she told me that the first time she wasn't successful in keeping the leadership, but after that she practiced and it went well. Sometimes you'll be more successful than other times, but don't forget it also takes time to learn a new language. Act like Marlies, who at first thought it wasn't possible, but didn't give up. You can do much more than you think you can. You will go on feeling miserable if you allow the negative little voices to determine your life. To learn to think realistically is the counter-charge. If you let your negative thoughts go, your feelings and also your (eating) behavior will change. Eventually you will become better at observing the chatter and return to the silence in yourself.

Exercise: dialogue with the Inner Saboteur.

Draw a vertical line across the middle of the page. On the left side write the comments of the inner saboteur and on the right side write your own answer as a rational thinker (true self). Don't let yourself be seduced into negotiating, because each compromise makes the inner saboteur stronger. You are in charge and so you have the last word, like Kathinka.

Learning to think differently

The way we think is essential for the choices we make.

Realistic thinking

Many statements from clients:

"Deep inside I don't really believe that I deserve to lead a happy and successful life."

"Something that goes well, can't keep on going well."

"Others, my work, study or other obligations are more important than taking care of myself."

"If I say no to others, they don't like me anymore."

"I believe that I will only be happy when I have the ideal figure."

"Each choice I make always leads me to a place where I don't want to be."

"I'm not worth investing time, money and energy in myself."

"Whatever I do, it is never good enough."

Our way of thinking has an enormous influence on our life. Recently I asked a woman on first acquaintance if she believed that she would ever get rid of her eating problem. She told me "No." Can you believe that years and years of therapy were not successful? If you are convinced that until your death you will be struggling with eating, then that will be true. You won't be successful in another way of dealing with eating as long as you let yourself be sabotaged in the way we have mentioned above and also in Chapter One. There is always a reason to maintain compulsive eating behavior. To recognize this process is the first step. The ideal situation would be that nothing is keeping you from healthy eating habits anymore, but the truth is that something like that, especially in the initial phase, requires a lot of attention.

> Marie: "I was scared when I found out that I had so many thoughts to sabotage myself with. It was painful to face, but, at the same time, I was aware that I had to let this form of self-sabotage go, to be able to realize my dreams. I understand better now why things went wrong in the past."

Constantly, I hear people wonder if they have enough willpower to leave their eating problem behind. Mental strength doesn't proceed so much from willpower, but basically from having insight and the right convictions. Your way of thinking has brought you to where you are now, but that same way of thinking doesn't bring you to where you would like to be. Thought-patterns are firm convictions, ideas, prejudices and opinions that we hold about ourselves and the world. We use them to filter out the things we don't want to see or hear. The way we talk to ourselves also determines the way we communicate with our environment. Problems will exist when we identify ourselves with meaningless, negative thought-patterns. Most of them have become a habit. If someone, for instance, is afraid to fail, he can believe that he "has to be perfect." That can subconsciously be used as a reason to do nothing, because it can provide the conviction that it cannot possibly succeed anyway. If we are unaware of this, it is possible that it will completely control us. That's why it is important to thoroughly investigate convictions that obstruct. If we let go of them one by one, it will have a deep influence on how we feel and how we behave. Every negative thought brings about negative physical reactions. It influences our digestion, we produce more adrenaline, our blood pressure rises, and so on. It is scientifically proven that negative thinking is a burden on our whole system. If we criticize ourselves constantly, in the long run we are going to hate ourselves. It is like a tape recorder playing the same negative tape in our head every day. This form of self-sabotage plays an important role in eating problems. Isn't it time to get rid of those worn-out tapes?

Many occurring irrational thoughts

Thoughts which have little to do with reality are irrational thoughts and are definitely not a help in the healing process. There are many forms of irrational thought. I hear many times from people with an eating problem:

The all-or-nothing principle (black/white thinking):

"I just ate too much, so the day is already spoiled and I might as well go on eating."

Fill-in thoughts for others and draw conclusions from them:

"He will think: what an ugly, fat and stupid girl. I believe he won't want to walk with me."

Generalizing:

"If my sister is not coming to my birthday party, probably the whole family isn't coming,"

Using double standards:

> "If I'm acting vulnerable I think it is weak, but if others do it, I think it is fine.

Stressing the negative side of an event and not seeing the positive side:

> "I felt so tired Saturday."
> (On inquiry it turned out that this woman felt very energetic the rest of the week, but she had completely forgotten that.)

Taking everything personally (being paranoid):

> "I enter the room and the conversation between two colleagues stops. Immediately I think they were talking in a negative way about me."

To put a label on yourself or others:

> "I'm not a fighter. I was destined to have an eating problem. It is because of my mother that I have an eating problem. She always forced me to clean my plate."

To take too much responsibility and condemn yourself:

> "It's my fault that he threw his back out."

Superstitious thinking:

> "As soon as the scales hit 130 pounds, everything in my life always goes wrong."

Reasoning emotionally:

> "I feel worthless, therefore I am worthless."

Presenting yourself and your environment with irrational demands:

"Until I am at my ideal weight I will allow myself only one meal a day."

"I am angry at my mother because she cooked the wrong things."

Exaggerating:

"Now that I finally had the courage to say no for once, I am afraid she won't want to see me anymore".

The thought-scheme

Event + Thoughts = Feelings + Behavior

Examination of irrational thoughts is of essential importance to bring you back to your true self. Your healing process goes more quickly when you are capable of realistic thinking. When someone says: "I like your hair," you must not ask yourself if it didn't look nice before; you must accept the compliment. You can no longer take everything to heart. And people who think differently from you are not monsters with whom you don't want to associate.

You can learn to get rid of negative convictions by being conscious of what you are actually thinking. Starting from there, you can create a new true reality, with the help of the following thought-scheme:

Describe briefly an event which gave you an unsatisfied and unwanted feeling. What were your expectations?

1. Put the automatic thoughts that went through your head, on paper.

2. Then challenge these thoughts with the help of the following questions:

- Are the things that I believe really true?

- What arguments support these thoughts?

- What arguments refute these thoughts?

- Is it in my interest to think this?

- Is it good for my health?

- What is my most important goal?

- Do I reach my goal with these automatic thoughts?

- What can I do to reach my goal?

- How do I feel when I imagine that I have reached my goal?

3. Describe briefly new realistic thoughts.

A reason can be a situation where you have strong negative emotions. Like Monique, who learns that Evelyn has successfully conquered her eating problem and thinks: "I won't succeed in getting rid of my eating problem."

Immediately she feels tense and sad and has the urge to "eat away" these feelings. With the help of the thought-scheme, she examined whether what she was thinking was right. When that didn't seem to be the case, the questions in the scheme helped her find new realistic thoughts and to experience more pleasant feelings. Here is her example:

1. **Automatic Thought**
"I will never succeed in getting rid of my eating problem."

2. **Challenge: Is it true?**
"I have made many attempts and nothing has helped. I don't believe in it anymore."

What are the arguments against these thoughts?
"If I think that nothing will help me to get rid of my addiction, then I will be stuck with it and I'm so tired of it. Evelyn told me that maybe I didn't use the correct strategy. She also struggled with this addiction for years and tried everything, but now she has been well for such a long time. If she is successful, maybe I can be successful. It is not in my interest to think negatively, it is not good for my health and I will never reach my goal if I think like that."

What is my most important goal?
"To be happy and have a normal eating pattern that goes with happiness."

Do I reach my goal with these automatic thoughts?
"No, if I keep on thinking like that, I won't be successful; I won't move forward."

What can I do to reach my goal?
"Evelyn told me that the way I think plays an important role in breaking through my binge eating. Thoroughly examining my thoughts is new to me. I will give this strategy a serious chance."

How will I feel when I imagine that I have reached my goal?
"Well, I have never thought about how that would feel [A moment later, after a fit of crying:] it is hard to put into words, but in any case I would feel intensely happy, powerful and peaceful."

3. **New realistic thought:**
   I trust myself.

Another example is Nancy, who has discovered that since she has begun to plan her meals and does not keep eating all day, her clothes fit better.

1. **Automatic thought:**
   I am afraid to lose weight, because, in the past, immediately after I lost weight, I gained weight again. So let me just start to binge eat again.

2. **Challenge: Is it true?**
   This is not an attempt simply to lose weight, but to discover a healthy way of life which in itself will lead to the loss of excess weight. To maintain this thought is not in my interest, certainly not beneficial to my health and with that kind of thinking I will absolutely not reach my goal.

   What is my most important goal?
   A healthy way of life

   Will I achieve my goal with these automatic thoughts?
   No, on the contrary.

   What can I do to reach my goal?
   Picking up the pieces and eating healthy and delicious meals at fixed times.

   How will I feel when I imagine that I have reached my goal?
   Relieved and free. [Nancy feels immediately relieved as soon as she realizes she is not on a diet]

3. **New realistic thought:**
   Through healthy eating I will get the figure that suits me.

Revealing thought patterns create clarity and freedom to choose.

It takes time to change deep convictions, but as soon as they give way to realistic thoughts, they deeply affect our behavior. This powerful technique is comparable to tools that remove weeds from our garden, and make room for beautiful flowers. Weeding regularly encourages our mind to feed itself with healthy thinking and living. That's why we will feel much better for the rest of our lives. Our thoughts create our lives!

> Nancy: I'm conscious now of the irrational thoughts that I told myself every day. By reading them again I think now: Did I say that to myself every day? No wonder I felt so miserable. More often now I put a hold on that stream of thoughts by saying to myself: STOP, I am doom-mongering again. I'm going to stop this. Because of this, I am able to handle this better all the time.

Exercise: realistic thinking

This is the thought-scheme given by Monique's and Nancy's examples: describe briefly a recent event where you had an unsatisfied and unwanted feeling. What were your expectations?

1. Write down the automatic thoughts you had immediately after, even if you do not think it makes sense. Keep the sentences short and simple.

2. Challenge these thoughts with the help of the following questions:

   • Are the things that I believe really true?

   • What arguments support these thoughts?

   • What arguments refute these thoughts?

   • Is it in my interest to think this way?

   • Is it good for my health?

   • What is my most important goal?

- Do I reach my goal with these automatic thoughts?

- What can I do to reach my goal?

- How do I feel when I imagine that I have reached my goal?

3. Try to write down new realistic thoughts.

If you are not satisfied with the result, then use other thoughts that are certainly true and really do help. Read once again the list of regularly occurring irrational thoughts. Find out if you have left something out.

- Do I really have proof that what I think is true, or do I have a tendency to fill in the picture like I have always done?

- What is reality?

- What is my reaction to such a thought?

- Is it good for me to keep this thought and what positive contribution could this thought make?

- Can I find one stress-free reason not to let go of this thought?

- Who or what would I be without this thought?

- What do I benefit if I should think about it differently?

- Are there other people who think completely differently about it? How can that be?

- What if someone whom I know well and whom I admire should produce counter-arguments?

- What would someone who doesn't care about weight and looks do in this situation?

Describe what you really see. Pay attention to words like: regularly, seldom, always, never, everyone, nothing, nobody, the men, the women. It is seldom black-and-white.

Replace words like "must" and "not allowed" and "cannot" by "maybe," "it is possible," "I aim at" and "I would like to see." Ask yourself if this thought will still matter in about ten or fifty years. In short, use your creativity to look at this situation and find a different way. If you keep a list of situations that bother you, track down your hidden convictions about yourself, your eating habits, controlling your weight, health, relationships, your body, and so on at a fixed time.

Challenge all the thoughts that sabotage your reaching your goal and replace them with new, realistic thoughts. Think also about the irrational thoughts that came into existence when you gave way to the partial-personalities [See the first exercise of this chapter].

To change your thought process is like learning a new language; it takes time and practice. Don't give in just because you are not always successful. Eventually, you will succeed. If you write down your irrational thoughts, the effect will be positive. Through this method you will learn more than learning by rote, because thoughts go by quick as lightning. We can settle them down by writing them down and then examining them. Just by writing them down time and again, you are taking a big step forward in your healing process. You can copy appendix 3.

Striking the balance

To feed yourself brings inner strength

Our attitude dictates how we experience our life

Sally: "My blood pressure was so high that my doctor ordered me to stop working. Suddenly, I realized that I was a living time-bomb. I ate away the stress of my job, just like all the other situations that I could not handle. I have been overeating for 25 years and was bursting at the seams. Because I was now confined at home by necessity and was confronted with myself, I realized that I didn't want to go on like this. It was now or never."

Elsa: "For years I have suffered from bulimia. I thought that I had it under control, but now that I am, according to everybody, much too skinny and I have been feeling very tense for quite some time, I worry about it. I want to feel happy again, but actually I don't want to gain weight. I'm scared of that. My mind tells me something has to happen, that's why I am here."

An eating problem is a continuing story in your life that influences your health, social contacts, the way you work and/or study, and so on. At a certain moment people reach the point where they can't go on any more in the old way. They have nightmares, become ill, get stuck in their studies or don't dare go to a party anymore. Such a crisis can lead to a fundamental change in their way of living, but it is also possible that people put up with it. It takes courage to travel down a new road.

It is not the problem itself, but the way we deal with it which defines how we experience our lives. It is the attitude that matters. The correct attitude is a crucial factor. There are people who desperately long for healing, but deep inside they don't believe there is a therapy that can help them. It is clear that this group won't reach its goal. The second category consists of people who are receptive to therapy, but still have some doubts.

As soon as they experience improvement, the healing takes place much more quickly.

The third group of people are those who completely open up and do what they have to do to be cured. They are prepared and convinced that therapy will support them through their inborn talent to heal. These different ways of thinking work on all the aspects of our lives.

When you answer the next questions on paper, you will get an impression of your attitude towards the question: will you keep on going the same old way or turn on to a new road?

To keep on going the same old way:

- What does it mean to you, if you don't change now and keep going the same old way?

- What advantages do you get from your eating problem?

- What will it deliver in two years?

- Are there different possible ways to reach what you like?

- What are the disadvantages of your eating problem?

- What disadvantages do you want to get rid of?

- What won't you have if you don't reach your goal?

- What is more important: temporary satisfaction that you have when you are binge eating, or feeling free and vital?

- What is the most important difference between your present situation and how you would like it to be?

- What do you think of the statement: when you do not make a decision now, you have decided to leave everything as it is?

Turning onto the new road:

- What makes it clear that you are now motivated to turn into the new road?

- Are you ready to invest time in yourself on a daily basis?

- When you believe that it is possible, how sure are you that you will succeed?

- What are your ideas about that?

- How would you know when you have reached your goal? What, for instance, have you gotten rid of?

- Which qualities do you need to reach your goal?

- What will it deliver in two years when you have reached your goal?

- Are you prepared to let go of old convictions about yourself, about your negative eating pattern?

- Are you prepared to take yourself by the hand with love?

- How does it feel to be in charge?

Are you capable of uttering the next sentences?

"It is possible to reach my goal."

"I deserve to reach my goal."

Now you know a little bit more about your motivation. I hope you want to turn onto the new road. If you are not sufficiently motivated yet, don't give up hope, but whenever you are ready for it, read this chapter again and do the exercises again.

Maybe certain things are still bothering you, like, "it has been there for so long," or, "I have already tried it so many times." It is possible that you did not apply the correct strategy. Ask for help from somebody you trust and who is serious about your problems. This person can think along with you. It might be too that you think that your situation is too complex: "I can't solve it myself, it is only possible with the help of a therapist." It may be true that you need specialized help with this, but ask yourself first if you are still looking for an excuse not to turn onto the road to healing. Again, the right attitude is a crucial factor!

From problem to goal

> Esmé: "Establishing concrete goals with little steps that seem realizable to me, gives me the feeling that I myself can set the tempo in the therapy."

It is evident that people who have realistic goals achieve much more than people who don't have them. The ones who write them down, achieve the most of all.

By writing down your goals and consciously making a decision, you are already on your way. This seems too good to be true. It has to do with four reasons:

1. Goals enhance your chances by the obligation you commit to.

2. Goals show that you are focused on solutions.

3. Goals stimulate you to give yourself completely.

4. Everything you do can be looked at in terms of your goal.

It removes you from your goal or it takes you closer to it. Our convictions have an important influence on our goals and on being successful. Change will only be successful when you dare to stick your neck out, by falling and getting up again. You can strengthen goals by remembering a successful experience. It is not important which experience as long as it was a successful one: getting your drivers license, for instance. What did you say to yourself then? How did you feel then? Revive the feeling that belongs to this successful memory.

In the first exercise, "the positive script," you wrote down what you wished your ideal life would look like. Hold on to that. Keep this picture in mind with the help of a collage, every night before going to sleep. If in your scenario you are regularly moving about, do so literally. If you regularly have contact with friends, take an active step. If in your scenario you spend time on hobbies, consider what you are going to start with. The next exercise is an important support.

Exercise: To set a goal

You will go from problem to goal by asking yourself: What would I like to have instead of . . . ?

What will your life be like if you have a healthy relationship with food?

What will you do? How will you look?

How will your environment react to this? Let go of your thoughts and feelings.

Then take the necessary steps in your mind. What is the first step?

Make an appointment with yourself that you are going to take the first step.

Let in the feelings raised by this decision.

When we write down our goals it is easier to realize them.

Write them down and read them to yourself. That way you give them more power and you will anchor them more and more in yourself.

Put the focus on what to you are the most important points of attention. [If necessary look back to the exercise "positive script".] Write in as much detail as possible a few of your goals for the next three months. No negatively worded goals like, "I'm not going to gorge," but positively worded goals like, "I enjoy eating three meals a day," of which one will be dinner. Keep in mind you must set realizable goals or you will disappoint yourself. The change should be a challenge, but also doable. Lack of self-esteem can be a reason that we are afraid of setting our goals too high, but don't bury your dreams! Our expectations dictate what we accomplish so you may have to change your convictions that stand in your way.

Formulate your goals in a way that you can later check if you have achieved them Preferably at a set time. For instance: this coming month I will go for a 45-minute walk at least five times a week.

Step 1: Next week I am going on a 30-minute walk every other day.

Step 2: The next week I'm going to walk for 30 minutes five times a week.

Step 3: Starting from week three I'm going to walk five times a week for 30 minutes.

With this you can use the next plan. You can copy appendix 4.

Goal: I want to achieve that . . .

Step 1: In a period of . . . to . . . I will do the following

Step 2: In a period of . . . to . . . I will do the following

Step 3: In a period of . . . to . . . I will do the following

Evaluation: Did I execute the step as I planned to ? Did I reach my goal with it?

If you have executed the steps as you have written them down and it didn't contribute to your goal, try to do it again and find out what or who can help you. Maybe your goal wasn't realistic enough. If you evaluate yourself daily you can

adjust your goals more easily. If again you are not successful, ask yourself, without blame, how that was possible. Find
the causes without being judgmental. Use your creativity to
reach your goal with another step. The person who is persistent will win.

In some cases, you may need someone to help you with a
persistent problem. Don't hesitate too long to find a therapist
who can help you with this.

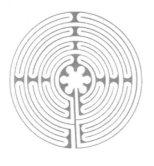

THE JOURNEY

3

MORE ENERGY

To come into contact with your real needs it is necessary to take time off to spend on yourself.

Taking better care of yourself

The only way to have time is to take time.

First refuel

This chapter offers suggestions on how to feel more energetic. An important advantage of this is that the need to gorge diminishes. There is one source of energy; the Chinese call it Chi, in India they call it Prana. That vitality you can find everywhere: in food, water, sunlight, but also in thoughts, emotions and in the drawing of our breath.

> Anika: "I don't know myself anymore. I'm exhausted, I do the things because of my willpower and I can cry about everything all day. In the past I used to gorge, but now I eat all day long. I know that this is not the solution. How can I break this vicious cycle?"

With new clients, as with Anika, almost all the time I hear that they feel exhausted. They have lost contact with their own feelings and needs, that's why, in time, physical as well as mental complaints have developed. Was it meaningful to work with Anika, who literally and figuratively was not comfortable with herself, emotionally

blocked?. Not in this phase: first we had to get her energy going
again. I offered some suggestions for her eating pattern and suggested she take food supplements like vitamins and minerals. [We
will talk about this in the next chapter.] We also talked about how
she could bring more structure into her everyday life. For people
who overeat compulsively, structure is essential. We need boundaries, we don't want (any longer) to get lost. If we are leading an
irregular life and there is no clear timetable, then we feel quickly
fatigued, irritated, emotionally unstable and we are less able to
make rational choices. Our biological clock becomes disturbed
and that will obviously have a negative effect on our eating behavior. We can bring structure in the form of a regular sleep-and-eat
rhythm, but also by planning time for relaxation on a daily basis.

To sleep and to wake

> Inez: "I started the day stressed. I stayed in bed for a while after
> the alarm clock rang and always had to hurry to get to work.
> In the car, on my way to the hospital where I work, I ate some-
> thing and as soon as I arrived, I kept on hurrying. After it was
> explained to me what the effect was of such a start to the day I
> decided to set the alarm clock to an earlier time. I get up qui-
> etly now and take the time to have breakfast at home. Such a
> relaxed start in the morning has an enormous influence on the
> rest of the day.

A good night's sleep is the basis of our mental and physical well-
being. Through stress and bad eating habits, our sleeping rhythm
can be disturbed, but habits also play a role in restless sleep or
insomnia. The latter I find constantly with people who demonstrate compulsive eating behavior. It is annoying that by sleeping
too long they feel more dazed and depressed. Most people need 6
to 8 hours of sleep. To sleep well is more important than to sleep
for a long time. That's why it is better to sleep for 6 hours uninter-

rupted than 9 hours with interruption. If we grant our body rest, the natural processes can repair themselves and the body will be in balance again. As I have said, sleeping a long time is no more than a habit. It is possible to have some problems in acquiring a new habit, but soon a new rhythm will develop. To give in too much to feeling tired, so that you sleep during the day, has a deleterious effect. Health psychologist Professor Jozien Bensing looked into this, and found that stress is a source of chronic fatigue, but the biggest problem, according to her, is that people who complain of chronic fatigue are sedentary. Her investigation in 2002 convinced her that this leads to a negative spiral effect instead of promoting healing.

To lie on the couch and drop all activities from your program is the worst possible reaction. Eventually this will make you more fatigued, weaker and without energy. The body is going to adjust physically to this lack of activity. Professor Bensing's conclusion: the person who acts like a delicate person, becomes a delicate person. According to her, when you suffer from chronic fatigue you should exercise twice a day for half an hour. Sleeping during the day is forbidden.

Tips for a good night's rest:

- After 8:30 in the evening no more strenuous work. In the hours before midnight you get the most rest. Try not to go to bed too late. If you are used to staying up late, move the time that you are going to sleep forward by half an hour every week.

- Try to go to bed at the same time every night as often as is possible and try to get up at the same time, even when you have a day off. That's how you keep your rhythm.

- It is a myth that sleeping in helps. It disturbs your rhythm and most people become more and more fatigued by it. You can catch up with sleep by going to bed earlier.

- Try to sleep without a sleeping aid. Quality sleep with sleeping aids is not healthy; it is addictive and a burden on your body. An alternative is possible by, for instance, visiting a homeopath or ortho-molec-ular dietician.

- Take a bath to which you have added calming-herbs (for instance lavender, fir or vanilla) a half hour before going to sleep. You can use this scent in the bedroom, too, in a little aroma burner, or put a few drops on your pillow.

- After this, drink warm herb tea (for instance cham-omile or valerian tea, or something similar.)

- Try to keep work-related material out of the bed-room. Try to do a relaxation-exercise [for instance the exercise "Strength of life" at the end of this chapter]. or use a CD with relaxation exercises or calming music on it.

- Electrical equipment can disturb your sleep. To be really sure, pull the plug out of the socket.

- The ten minutes after you fall asleep and the first ten minutes after you wake up have a strong influ-ence on your subconscious. So just before going to sleep try to avoid watching TV or having difficult conversations. It is better to read a relaxing book.

- If it is impossible to fall asleep, put a warm hot-water bottle on your stomach or at your feet.

- Do recurrent annoying dreams bother you? Say to yourself a couple of times at the moment that you are ready to go to sleep, " I want to have a dreamless sleep now and want to wake up feeling rested and relaxed," or, "Tonight I expect to have a beautiful, relaxing dream."

- Do you want to learn to remember your dreams? Chapter 7 tells you how you can learn that.

- Concentrate on your breathing until you fall asleep.

Tips for waking up and resting during the day:

- Get up early and always at the same time, even though occasionally you may have gone to bed late. That will keep your rhythm.

- The first ten minutes after waking up are very important. Your subconscious is especially vulnerable then to negative as well as positive suggestions.

- In the morning, take your time so that you will start your day relaxed. The beginning of the day often determines our state of mind for the rest of the day.

- Never skip breakfast. In the next chapter I will elaborate on this.

- Exercise when you are feeling dull, plan relaxation moments and, if needed, go to bed early.

- If you are sleepy and can't keep your eyes open during the day, limit yourself to the "power nap." That means twenty minutes rest. No longer, because otherwise you will end up in a different sleep phase. Rest only if you are extremely exhausted.

- Don't exhaust yourself during the day, but consciously take moments of rest. Then you will sleep better at night.

Make time for relaxation

Mary, a new client, protested when I suggested that she should do relaxation exercise at home on a regular basis. She told me that she did not have the time for that, because her life was very busy. She gave herself no rest and had trouble making choices, always afraid of making a mistake. During the session it became clear to her that an attack of binge eating is often a sign of an underlying need: now it is my turn and I will put myself first.

Most women demand a lot of themselves. They want to look good, meet friends, have a nice job and at the same time raise children and keep their love life at a certain level, and so on. Making room for relaxation on a daily basis is a necessity for a healthy way of life. I advise clients to set aside at least half an hour for themselves every day, time during which you don't have to do anything. Do what you like to do at that moment: read, take a bath, listen to your favorite music, go for a walk outdoors or enjoy a relaxation exercise. So instead of occupying ourselves with food, we can learn to feed ourselves in a different way. The only way to experience inner peace is to create a certain amount of discipline in our lives.

The Dalai Lama says: "You must discipline yourself to feel happy. In that way we no longer feed the things that are not really a part of us, but we choose the things we love."

An important part of relaxation is breathing. To breathe is to live! When we inhale we experience life and energy, while through exhalation we can let go and rest.

When we are stressed, the natural rhythm of breathing changes, from low and slow to high and fast. Because of this we are inhaling less oxygen, don't feel fit and start to breathe even more quickly and shallower. Through breathing exercises we can calm a restless mind, but also feel more energetic. A full breathing flow brings space and comforts the body by purifying the waste materials. Rhythmical breathing also brings the two halves of the brain in balance.

Tips to relax:

- Create your own retreat in which you can leave the things behind in order to "refuel."

- Nature has a relaxing effect. For instance, take a walk or ride your bike.

- If your energy increases it is important to use it sparingly. Don't use it up immediately.

- Plan your activities for the day. Avoid boredom, but be careful not to do too much. Take regular breaks to rest so that you don't become exhausted. Keep in mind that exhaustion can easily lead to binge eating.

- If you think it is difficult to relax, don't hesitate to look for help with this. As personal therapy you can choose breathing therapy, for instance, or haptonomy. In groups you can practice yoga or qi gong.

- Singing is a direct way to better breathing and feeling energetic.

Exercise: vitality

You can do this exercise while sitting, standing or lying. Close your eyes and concentrate on your breathing without changing it. Imagine that with each exhalation, stress, fatigue and things like that disappear into the ground through a little trapdoor under your feet.

After you have concentrated on the exhalation a few times, try to imagine that when you inhale, healing energy is streaming through the top of your head, to the depths of your being. You can also try to send energy to a spot in your body that needs extra care. You can do this exercise several times a day in stressful periods. It is also an ideal relaxation exercise when you can't sleep.

Increasing vitality

*Meditation is one of the shortest ways
to inner peace and vitality.*

Meditation

> Ilona: "Since I started meditating on a daily basis, I am more
> capable of observing situations instead of letting my emotions
> run away with me."

Meditation is a powerful method to bring us in contact with the
person that we really are. Some people immediately start to think
of vague trivialities. That's a pity; because meditation is primarily
a way for you to concentrate on finding peace. Some people think
that meditation involves sitting in an uncomfortable lotus position while thoughts keep running through your head. That picture
is not correct. Consciously concentrating on one thing, giving all
your attention for instance, to doing the dishes, is actually a form
of meditation.

As children, we did this by looking attentively at the moon or
studying the clouds while we were lying on the grass. Meditation
can help you appreciate everyday beauty by paying attention to the
here and now. In Japan, flower arrangements and the art of archery
are a form of meditation. In other Eastern countries, sitting to

meditate is customary, while in China meditative movement (qi gong) is very popular. We are not used to consciously being present in the here and now, because our minds are constantly distracted by all kinds of things. Through meditation we bring all parts of ourselves together again to make us whole. We turn back to our centre and thus learn to understand ourselves. By meditating regularly we become more and more conscious of the silent witness in ourselves. It is that loving part that we can look upon as an inner compass that gives direction to our lives. Many physical complaints that come from stress, like headache and back pain, can decrease or disappear through meditation. It is an important key to a balanced eating-and-living pattern. We learned this through hundreds of studies that have been done worldwide. The prominent ayurvedic doctor and philosopher, Deepak Chopra, known throughout the world as a pioneer in the area of the connection between body and mind, refers to this in his books.

His experience has always been that when someone has reverted to addictive behavior, it seems they have stopped meditating. He looks at meditation as the most effective technique to cure addiction of any kind.

Positive effects of meditation are:

- It brings inner peace, vitality and strength.

- It diminishes fear.

- It makes it easier to overcome addictive behavior.

- It makes you more creative.

- It makes you more youthful.

- Emotional instability diminishes (the nervous system has a chance to rest).

- Destructive thinking patterns diminish.

- It improves health (strengthens, among other things, the immune system, regulates the hormones and has a favorable effect on metabolism).

- It strengthens the ability to concentrate.

- It promotes inner growth by allowing contact with your true self.

Very often I hear people say that they can't stop thinking, but thoughts are a part of meditation. If we let thoughts come and go, by just looking at them, our mind can rest. However, in the initial phase most people with an eating problem are very restless; they can hardly sit or lie still to do a relaxation exercise or to meditate. So it is often much easier to empty your mind by doing a visualization.

After a visualization of a favorite little retreat, Martha said:

"I was at my favorite little place where as a child I liked best to hide. This was a little hut I had put together at the end of our dead-end road. I'm so glad that I have the ability to visit this little retreat when I wish to. Here I feel safe and find myself again."

This visualization exercise is described at the end of this sub-chapter.

You can also work with meditative movement-forms like tai-chi, aikido or chi-neng. These meditative movement-forms focus on promoting body-mind integration. I look upon them as the cement that connects body and mind. During the consciousness training, Samantha discovered the value of chi-neng.

"When I got home from work I didn't know what to do with myself. Many times I felt very restless and I was preoccupied with food. When I get home now the first thing I do is practice chi-neng. That brings peace and energy."

This simple art of movement is focused on developing your inner strength, stability, personal growth and on keeping you in good shape. It was developed by Dr. Pang Ming especially for seriously ill people, and it can be done easily at home. The Chinese government has recognized it as the best healing form of qi gong. By doing this for 20 minutes a day, you will quickly experience a reduction of stress and an increase in energy.

A little while after I had encountered chi-neng, I discovered that this form of qi gong was exactly what I was looking for. To my astonishment, within a short time my chronic complaints had disappeared. For years my body was a hated opponent, but now, thanks to chi-neng, I pay attention to it every day in a loving way.

Tips for meditation:

- Discipline helps us to turn inward. Try to spend twenty minutes a day on meditation.

- Meditate in a place where you know you are not going to be disturbed, because silence is an essential requirement to re-energize yourself.

- Meditate always at the same time of day, so that it becomes a habit. Meditation in the morning will ensure that your day will start in calmness. When you meditate after an active day, it will help you to clear your mind.

Experience the meditative working of nature by, for instance, taking a walk in silence. Being out in a natural setting, you can find yourself experiencing silence and harmony. Concentrate on your breathing without changing it at all. When your mind wanders, lead it back.

Exercise

Exercise is a step towards change, progress and renewal. Clients who don't exercise have all kinds of excuses. The "limited self" likes to have attention. Again, discipline is needed here, just as with meditation. Start to exercise, but do this slowly; not the "all-or-nothing" approach, where you risk dropping out. Exercise daily for 30 minutes minimum, but preferably for three-quarters of an hour. According to Harm Kuipers, a former world champion ice skater and professor of Kinetics, this will have a positive effect on your health.

Exercise rests your mind and gives you more energy and physical and psychological balance. Further, your body can get rid of stress hormones. That's why exercise is a perfect natural remedy for stress and fatigue. After a while, you are going to like it. Activities you like are the most effective.

Leonie: "I was addicted to exercising. Next to vomiting it was my way to lose weight. In the end I could hardly move because of the pain. If I couldn't exercise for two hours a day I punished myself by not eating. Finally, I became very ill and couldn't visit the fitness centre anymore. Now I have learned to listen to my body and discover bit by bit what I like to do."

Don't overdo: choose a form of exercise that suits you. Perhaps you feel like taking a walk, riding your bike (or stationary bike), skipping rope, swimming, dancing, or walking on the treadmill while you sing to music or watch a movie. There are videos for sale with exercises you can do at home. Exercise in a way that you won't get short of breath: that is not the point. Vary the exercises, so that you use different groups of muscles. It happens often that people who think they are too fat, or really are too fat, underestimate the effect of active exercise and put the emphasis on a drastic reduction of calories. The trap is that strict dieting can lead to binge eating.

Also, it is possible that by eating less we could gain weight because of a slowing down of the metabolism. This could be compared to an open fire: to keep the fire going, we have to throw a log on it once in a while. Of course it is important to pay attention to what we eat: vegetables, fruit, whole grain products, as unprocessed as possible. Along with that, we must activate the metabolism by exercising daily.

> Carrie: "I always hated to exercise. It was not for me. But now I have discovered that I like it because I no longer look at it as something I have to do. I feel much more comfortable in my body and with myself. I miss it when I don't exercise even for a day. It is also a "exhaust-valve" for frustrations. Awhile ago I was angry at someone. Suddenly, I noticed that on the tread-mill I could work off my aggression. In the past I would have automatically eaten it away."

A list of the most important reasons to exercise:

- It activates the immune system.

- It prevents health problems (heart and vascular dis-ease, osteoporosis, and diabetes. Also when you exercise enough, there is less chance of stomach and breast can-cer).

- Helps to normalize the working of insulin, which is important for problems with the blood sugar level.

- curbs an excessive appetite.

- Improves your physical fitness.

- Increases energy.

- Helps to remove waste (stimulates, among other things, the working of the intestines).

- Helps one to become grounded, to connect with the earth.

- Lessens stress-related symptoms.

- Helps mental relaxation.

- Improves the mood (manufactures the "happiness hormone" endorphin).

- Strengthens the digestion and burns fat.

- Slows down the process of bone decalcification.

- Improves sleep rhythm.

- Builds self-confidence.

Tips on exercising:

- To exercise daily for three quarters of an hour is more effective than doing it once for two hours and skipping it the following day. The advantage of this is that you can integrate it easily into your everyday life.

- Make room every day for physical exertion and make sure that you can rest afterward if necessary.

- If you are overweight, exercise more than twenty minutes, because only then will the fat start to burn.

- The Health Counsel especially advises people who do sedentary work to exercise for at least half an hour a day to keep their weight down.

- If you exercise with a friend, there is more chance that you will do it faithfully.

- Muscular pain can occur if you are training too stringently, or in the wrong way, or with new exercises. Don't overdo: if you are training certain groups of muscles, you have to let them rest for 24 or 48 hours, but don't sit down, keep moving.

- You will only really profit from exercising when it becomes a regular part of your life-style, but to exercise more you must really want it. Examine your irrational thoughts about exercise, challenge them and replace them with rational thoughts.

- Take care that exercising is not going to lead to an excessive, compulsive activity. It happens very often that one addiction can lead to another. Too much exercise is as bad as too little.

Exercise: Your little place in nature

Close your eyes and concentrate on your breathing without changing it. Next, picture yourself somewhere in a natural setting (real or imagined) where nobody can come without your permission. The temperature is pleasant. Take the time to look at the surroundings, which colors, forms and sounds most attract you. What does it mean to you to be here? How do you feel? Take time to enjoy this place fully and to recharge yourself. Go back regularly in your mind to this little natural retreat.

Energy gluttons and energy givers

We keep on longing for food until
we know how to fulfill ourselves.

The consumption-society

> Karina: "On the one hand I want peace and quiet on the week-
> end, to relax from my work and just enjoy my husband and
> baby at home, but at the same time I'm afraid to miss some-
> thing, so the result is that I still have a full weekend agenda."

In the first chapter I wrote about inner emptiness. The consumption-society likes to hook into this. By continually seeking
pseudo-satisfaction, we are constantly restless and, in the long run,
we become literally and figuratively over stimulated and out of balance. Not only do certain contacts and obligations use up a lot of
energy, but wanting to do too many enjoyable things is a trap. It is
not realistic to hold on to all those activities in a society with unlimited possibilities. We exhaust ourselves and lose our ability to heal.
It is temping to blame this madness on the consumption-society.
But we "hunger" because we are cut loose from our true feelings.
Many people think they will be happy only when they are slender,
or have found that great partner, or gotten that super job, but when
that is accomplished, after a short while they become restless again

and the next need has to be satisfied. They are so busy hunting for their ideal, that they will remain unfulfilled.

Deep inside, people are afraid that they will get bored; they are scared of the emptiness. They try to avoid loneliness and not only with the aid of food. The inner critic will always find something to worry about, will try to control us, but is basically unfulfilled. When our life is dominated by this saboteur, we are living in a very small world. When we lose ourselves and are secluded from the world, we can feel like a lost child. Many people long to be satisfied with what they have, but they don't know how to make that adjustment.

The saboteur is searching for fulfillment outside itself, but doesn't know it can only be found within itself. Not outside ourselves will we find the source of satisfaction, fulfillment and joy, but in ourselves. We can find this source by turning inward. Then we'll see the forest and not only the trees.

To develop enough activities

Compulsive eating behavior is going to go on until we know how to fulfill ourselves. My father was someone who realized that he had to find happiness in himself. The volatile consumption-society could go to blazes as far as he was concerned. He was a gifted man, with many interests. Nature was a huge source of inspiration to him, providing him with many unusual hobbies that he could totally wrap himself up in. That was the way he fed himself. Through him, I discovered how important hobbies are and how you can start to enjoy yours:

- It should be something you choose of your own will, that you can do alone and that you would like to do almost every day.

- It should not take much effort, and since you enjoy it, there is no self-criticism here.

- It should have a certain value for you.

When eating is your most important "hobby" or the only thing you enjoy, you have a problem, because your enjoyment can last only a little while. To eat in a different way to conquer binge eating is not enough. You have to deal with changing your life and develop fulfilling activities. To be active is important, so you should not do something passive like watching TV. Seclude yourself from the world. Warn your housemates and, if necessary, turn off the phone. Focus all your attention on your activity and try not to allow any thought that will distract you. If you don't know what activity you are interested in, ask yourself what you liked to do in the past. You can also record in a diary those moments when you felt the happiest. In this way you can discover what is the most suitable activity for you. Or you can imagine yourself expressing your inner life in a creative way.

Maybe you see yourself playing music, writing, drawing, singing, designing clothes, dancing, making jewelry or taking photos. It doesn't matter what it is as long as you have the feeling that it gives you energy and fulfillment. Things that are realized exist first in our imagination. So if you begin to fantasize for a little while over the different possibilities, it often seems that suddenly you are doing things that suit you.

What do I need?

> Ilona: "Day and night I was there for my family and for the people at work. I was also the one who could not say no when my parents called upon me. I was empty; the only thing I could enjoy was French cheese and bread. I had nothing more to give. I'm learning now for the first time to stand up for my own needs and that that is not egotistic. I feel now that I'm of use to my environment when first I take good care of myself. For years I lived my life on automatic pilot, but now I have the feeling that my life has really begun."

Ilona has a family with three children and thought that it was egotistic to put herself first, but would it be good for her environment if she collapsed? An eye-opener to her was the comparison with the safety rules in an airplane. When the cabin pressure falls, we have to put an oxygen mask on ourselves before we are able to help the children. If Ilona doesn't take good care of herself, how will she be able to function properly and be there for her family? This example gave her the strength to consciously put herself first.

It is essential for the energy of your household that you take good care of yourself. That means to make and keep contact with what you really like to do and make time for that. By noting what brought energy and what took energy away, Ilona found out that she wanted to change. Very soon she realized that for years she had wanted to quit her job. She applied elsewhere and was hired immediately. She set definite times to be with her husband and children. She makes time daily, too, for at least one energy-giving activity to recharge herself completely. After a month Ilona said that the magic of compulsive eating had faded. "I'm living again!"

Ilona shows us that when we discover what we need and give it to ourselves, the searching outside ourselves will come to an end.

Tips for more energy:

- If you write down your daily activities for two weeks, you will get a picture of what uses up energy and what brings energy. Ask yourself critically if certain activities are necessary. Can't you do it differently or let someone else do it?

- Make a list of things that energize you. Often they are the smallest things. If you can't come up with anything pleasant, think back to what you liked to do as a child. For example, as a child, Manon liked to color. Now she is coloring her handmade mandalas.

- Find your irrational thoughts about which things bring energy and which take energy away from you, and let go of them.

- There are givers and takers. Your energy will improve when you pay attention to people who energize you. Watch out for your own "taking-tendency."

- Did you know that being constantly nice to others can be addictive too? Being nice to yourself is the most important thing you can do.

- Start cutting back on your personal obligations to friends and acquaintances (like birthday parties). Don't make appointments with people out of pity or when you don't feel like it.

- If you say no, keep to that. Don't let yourself be seduced by having to defend yourself.

- Being fatigued is a signal to rest; pay attention to this signal. Although you don't feel fatigued, still take a rest at consciously chosen moments.

Feeling blue, feeling good

Isabel told me that since last week she had been in a "dip" again and didn't know how to get out of it. I asked her what her recipe was. She looked at me in astonishment and then had to laugh. Below are the main ingredients for getting into a "dip"—that is:

- Working too hard, studying too hard and doing too many odd jobs within a specific period of time (or at least 2 of the 3).

- Think negatively and aim at perfection.

- Never say "no."

- Suppress all your feelings.

- Stand on the scales every day.

- Help everyone as much as is possible and do nothing that you like to do.

- Put on clothes that are too small.

- Add a little pound of stress, compulsive eating and too much alcohol.

- If you reach the boiling point, you will sink away into days of apathy, doing nothing, and your depression is at hand.

I told Isabel that I thought it was a perfect recipe to feel fatigued and miserable. She realized that she was attached to sorrow, that she had come to rely on it. I thought her statement was striking: "I have to hit bottom first and then get up from there again." That was her conviction for years and until now she had held onto it. By challenging this irrational thought she got a different look at it. Next I asked her: "What is your recipe to get out of that "dip?" Here is her "out-of-the-dip" recipe:

- Alternate boring activities with pleasant ones, because you are worth it.

- Set reasonable goals and stick to them.

- Get enough rest.

- Replace irrational thoughts with realistic ones.

- Enough is good enough.

- Dare to say no. Don't promise things you can't live up to.

- Look at exercise as a daily pleasure.

- Talk about your feelings.

- Throw away the scale and trust the feeling about how your clothes fit you.

- Only wear clothes in which you feel comfortable.

- Drink at least 8 glasses of water a day and eat healthy food.

- Admit it if you can't do something on your own, ask for help.

Isabel said: "I'm okay too when I ask for help, with that I'm giving something to the other person as well." She realized that she only got out of her "dip" when she talked about her feelings. To feel the emptiness is to fill the emptiness.

After I asked Isabel how she managed to get herself in a "dip," I began to ask every client to write down her "secret" recipe. Through this exercise they not only realize how they let themselves slide back, but they also acknowledge that they are able to go on with their lives again much more quickly than in the past. The challenging of irrational thoughts and the expression of feelings are essential to feeling love for ourselves.

Exercise: your "in/out-of-the-dip" recipe

What does your "in/out-of-the-dip" recipe look like? Write it down and if necessary hang it somewhere in sight so that you will be reminded of it regularly.

Soul food

We will only be happy if we feed our soul
as much as our body.

A little diary for happiness

Instead of sitting in the dark, we can just put on the light. I have mentioned that people with an eating problem tend to concentrate on what is not perfect.

It is time now for a few suggestions to help us have another look at ourselves and our environment. First we can do this by keeping a diary of positive experiences, so that we can see the things that are good and that are making us happy. Veronique wrote about this:

> "At the end of every day I write down the beautiful moments in my little happiness diary. Because of that, I live a more conscious life and I realize that there are many moments in my daily life to be thankful for. This little book revived my optimism and it makes me feel very rich. My sister is going through a difficult time, so recently I gave her a little happiness diary. The next day she told me that I was yesterday's moment of happiness, because I gave her something that brightened her life."

Eating problems are keeping us away from the here and now, because we are constantly preoccupied with food—in our mind or in reality. We can experience fulfillment by being present in the moment, so that we can hear the birds' song, see a friend's smile and feel what that means to us.

We can feel the sun on our face or the wind blowing through our hair. We can set ourselves right by not giving way to traumatic circumstances, but also by paying attention to the moments of joy. Keeping a little happiness diary shows us that even in difficult times there are moments to be thankful for.

It is often hidden in little things. In Hawaiian the word "thanks" means "to bless" as well as "to give power." This little diary has another important goal.

One remembers the failures more easily and longer than the successes. That's why we have a picture of ourselves that is too negative. Even our upbringing adds to that. I read somewhere that until we are twelve years old, for each "yes" we hear seventeen "no's." If every day we look back on the day for a happy moment that we can record in our little diary, our self-confidence will rise. Buy yourself a beautiful little book in which you write for yourself only, mentioning for instance the compliment you got or how you dared to say what was bothering you. Write about a task that you finished or the things you did during the day that were successful. Maybe you enjoyed a moment of relaxation or a walk in the park. When there is a time that you can't think of anything, read carefully what you wrote the day before. In the beginning, it can feel strange to note only things that are positive. That's why I suggest that, at first, clients write down one positive occurrence a day. Very soon they will find many positive things in a day.

This way they begin to feel that negative occurrences have less influence on their lives. Many clients tell me that after some time, they become more aware and perceptive and think, "This makes me happy, I am going to write that down later."

I keep it in my night stand and write in it before I go to sleep.

Although in the beginning there may be only one sentence on the page, it still has a positive effect and brings fulfillment in the here and now.

Being open to appreciation

Betty could see very well the qualities of the people around her, but absolutely not the qualities in herself. So I asked her to write down her own qualities. At the next session, Betty told me that for an hour she had sat there with a piece of paper in front of her, and all that came up were negative thoughts and disapproval. People with an eating problem tend to emphasize only things that are not good about them. That is not realistic. I told Betty to ask a few people who know her well if they would put into words what qualities they think she has. She asked her husband and her almost grown-up daughters. She wrote in her little happiness diary:

> "Enthusiastically, all three of them answered my question. One put it into words and looked me right in the eye; the other wrote it down for me with a golden pen, so that those words would never be lost again. I was crying with joy; I could hardly believe that they were talking about me, the warmth that came from them was indescribable. I'm sure it is sincere— they love me, It gives me a lot of strength, it is becoming more and more a part of myself. I believe now that I have these qualities. It make me strong and I can learn to love myself."

Another example is provided by Maria. Previously she had told me that she would ask her mom what she thought about her, but that she believed her mother would react in a negative way. That was her interpretation and I told her so. I asked her if she was willing and able to let go of her negative anticipation and to ask her mother if she wanted to talk about her qualities. The next time she came in she told me that it had worked out very positively and that the paean of praise had touched her deeply.

You, too, can ask a few loving people to tell you what they value in you. Take the compliments and write them in your little happiness book.

The wise guide

> Kim: "I was ill and for a couple of days I felt pitiful and alone. Although friends visited me, I missed the arm around my shoulders. A man who would be there only for me. I made a fool of myself eating, because now when I was pitiful and alone I was allowed to eat everything. At a certain moment I started to do a visualization exercise. I imagined that I was at my favorite little rustic spot. Suddenly in this picture an old unknown man appeared. He was friendly but decisive, as he made it clear to me that I had to pull myself out of this self-created swamp. His appearance made such an impression on me that I was promptly able to pull myself together."

There is a part of us that still is connected with oneness, connected with our true self. This wise and skilled part knows what to do and what not to do. It is a part of a never-ending field of power and appears to us in different ways, through body-sensations, but also through dreams and pictures and memories that suddenly well up. Because of this unknown man, Kim looked at herself differently. In contrast to her inner saboteur this wise guide seemed to offer a friendly, helpful hand.

Right after she told me about that experience, Kim came up with a question. She had to decide whether to go on with her present work project or stop it and start a different one. Both options seemed attractive to her and she didn't know the best thing to do. I suggested that she open herself to this figure again. She came in contact with him again through a visualization and that's how she succeeded in making a decision. We don't have to do it on our own. When we are asking for "higher" intervention, we can take a step back and allow ourselves symbolically to take the hand of a guide, guardian angel or God. Guides give advice, but don't force us to do anything. When we fully open up to this help, we can get answers that we could not think of ourselves.

Exercise: meeting a wise person

Go to your favorite retreat and make sure that you won't be disturbed! Put on some relaxing music. Take time while you are resting to experience the following visualization:

Imagine that you are in a valley. The sky is blue, the sun is shining and there is a cool breeze. Enjoy the mountainous surroundings and open up to the colors, the fragrances, the forms and sounds. You see a variety of blooming flowers. Imagine you lose your usual worries. Take time to feel contact with the earth. Something in you makes you decide that you are going to climb the tall mountain you see before you. You are walking through the forest inhaling the delicious fir-fragrance, hearing the rustle of the wind and the chirping of the birds. You are climbing between the trees and you notice that you are going higher.

Then the path becomes steeper. You feel the power of your body streaming pleasantly through you. It becomes quieter around you. You notice that the air is fresher and thinner. The climbing is more difficult. But you keep going, because you feel a deep longing to reach the top of the mountain. You can see it more and more clearly. You look down and can see the deep valley with a single little village.

Now you reach the top of the mountain, which is on a large plateau. The sky is deep blue and it is incredibly quiet.

In the far distance you can see someone who radiates a lot of love, wisdom and light. He or she notices you and you walk towards each other. This wise person smiles at you and you feel a deep affection coming from this figure. Now you are standing opposite each other and you look him or her in the eye. Spontaneously, you hold out your hands. You feel that with all your heart you open yourself to the light that he or she radiates. You refresh yourself with this. This wise guide invites you to sit. You can ask all the questions you want to ask. You listen attentively to the answers.

After a while you say goodbye to the guide. You have learned that you are always welcome and the wise figure hands you a present. It is an object from which you can get power.

Take everything that you have experienced with you consciously to your daily life, where there is always room for change and insight. Start to breathe more deeply, return to your retreat and do some stretches. As you do this visualization often, you will notice that the quality of the wise figure will manifest itself more and more in you. The guide can show itself in different shapes, depending on the help you need. It is possible that you will experience only a fluid presence or a diffuse impression of colors. The wise figure communicates through symbols or feelings. If you don't get an immediate answer, it may come later in the day or in a dream. At a later stage (sometimes it happens spontaneously), you can imagine that you fuse with this wise figure and that you are the wise one that is free and radiating. It lets you look through his or her eyes at yourself and the environment. From a never-ending perspective you look around you filled with compassion.

You can tape this text and listen to it when you need it. You can also do this visualization together with someone else. One guiding the other.

4

THE DIFFERENT DIMENSIONS OF FOOD

---

*If you have leaned to still emotional hunger
with something other than food, your physical
hunger will no longer be threatening.*

Back to the basics

When we let ourselves be led by our true selves, then we are listening to the nutritionist that lives in each of us.

Filling or feeding

Although good nutrition is essential to healing, during the consciousness training there is no emphasis on eating. There we limit ourselves to treating the symptoms.

The substance of the matter is to find oneself again. But then again,, we can't achieve healing, without doing just what people with eating problems are afraid of, that is, to eat. By eating, they meet fears and they can find out what they are struggling with. During the training we focus on eating behavior, not only by talking about it, but also by letting the women feel, in a non-threatening way, what it does to them. The one who is afraid of getting fat is an easy target to go on a crash diet. Many people, however, start to binge eat when there are problems in sight. That's why they can't stick to their diet and it becomes a vicious cycle. Because of the "yo-yo effect," our metabolism slows downs which can result in weight gain. We can think that binge eating will go away all by itself, we can go on counting calories, or search for the next diet, or a different therapist, but for those who want lasting results it means "back to the basics."

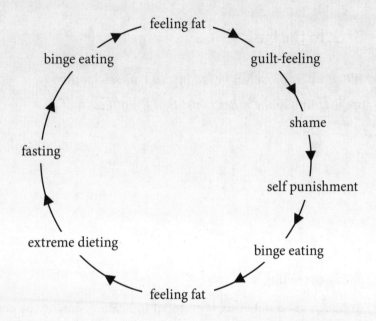

That means, next to daily exercises, healthy, moderate and varied eating. The more often we introduce tasty, healthy food into our lives, the easier it becomes to say no to "fillers" like candy and salted crackers. But if you choose to, indulge yourself, make sure you enjoy such a moment intensely. Take time for it, focus on what you are eating and accept the possible consequences. To change our lifestyle doesn't mean we are never again allowed to eat something sweet or high in fat. I don't believe in extreme eating habits, because the problem with extremes is they threaten to control our lives. That's how one eating problem can be replaced by another kind of eating problem: fixation on healthy food (orthorexia).

As soon as we label a certain food product as good or bad, we cut ourselves off from signs that our body can give us about the things we eat. By listening to this we can discover what really feeds us. Give yourself time to get used to a "back to the basics" eating pattern. To lose weight or to gain weight is not important in this phase, it is important now that you discover how much food your body needs in different situations and what you feel comfortable with. If, for instance, you eat a lot of heavy food, you don't suddenly change your eating pattern. What happens first is that the perception changes. The full-to-overflowing stomach no longer offers a solution. Gradually you leave the old pattern behind and learn to trust the wisdom of your body.

> Brigitte: "Before I started the training I allowed myself to eat only fruit, lettuce and yogurt. Now I plan a week's menu, cook only for myself and eat a variety of foods. I started to realize that my old eating pattern actually caused me to crave delicious 'forbidden' things."

What I often notice with clients is their one-sided eating habits. If you have no control over your life, at least you can control your weight and eating habits. However, this can in turn trigger an eating binge. This binge eating pattern often consists of calorie-rich food that normally we forbid ourselves to eat. Eating a well-balanced diet is not only important to prevent binge eating, but it is also important to supply enough of the essential nutrients. The body also becomes lazy if we continually eat the same food. In real life it seems that planning meals in advance helps to bring more variety to our eating pattern, and gives us something to hold onto. The struggle we have with food is the struggle we have with ourselves. It is important to be freed from old habits and, not to mention, from the pleasures which keep us imprisoned. We can only leave our eating problem behind after we have developed self-awareness. By finding out the reasons why we eat when we are not hungry, we can let go of our compulsive eating behavior one step at a time. It starts with taking the time to observe ourselves every day.

To love yourself starts with observing yourself. The path to inner freedom challenges us to become an observer. Then we can join ourselves with something that is bigger than ourselves, and then we will be capable of doing a lot more.

Digesting

In our lives, literally and figuratively, we have to stow away a lot. And in terms of food we have to stow away a lot, too. If we overload our washing machine, the laundry will not get clean. The same thing applies to our stomach. If we stuff ourselves with food, the digestive tract will not function properly and there will be a problem. Also, the excessive consumption of junk food, loaded with artificial ingredients, can lead to fatigue, irritability and intolerance of certain food. Not only what we eat, but how we eat, is important. Stress holds back the production of digestive enzymes and juices so that this food is not sufficiently digested and absorbed. Our body is then not able to get enough proteins and minerals from the food, which can lead to fatigue and gastrointestinal problems. Chewing influences the digestion and the absorption of nutrients. Chewing is also a natural way of releasing aggression. During a binge eating attack, hardly anything is tasted and there is hardly any chewing, but both are essential to alleviating hunger. A good digestion is not only important for food, but also for life experiences. Then we absorb what we can use and eliminate what is not useful. If we are capable of digesting sufficiently what is on our plate, we prevent our carrying with us the unprocessed remains with all of their consequences. I will go into this in more detail in chapter 6.

The value of breakfast

Are you afraid of immediately starting to eat too much in the morning or don't you give yourself enough time to eat breakfast? It can be tempting to stay in bed longer and leave the house without breakfast, because many people think they save calories that way. It is also possible that you are not hungry in the morning, often because of a disturbed eating rhythm. If you are eating late at night, you are likely to feel full in the morning. You can break through this pattern by starting the morning with a good breakfast and not eating anything after eight o'clock at night.

Good reasons to eat breakfast:

- Morning and afternoon are the best times for burning off your food. Skipping meals like breakfast on a regular basis, can cause the body to burn less food, so that you gain weight more quickly. Research shows that the person who wants to lose weight should especially not skip breakfast. If you eat breakfast, the chance of gaining weight becomes considerably less.

- You activate your bowel movements.

- Binge eating attacks often occur because of neglected hunger signals. By not skipping breakfast or lunch you will have less tendency to snack later in the day. Feeling hungry is the most important reason for reaching for a quick, often fattening, snack.

- Various research has shown that if you eat breakfast, you have less chance of a disturbed metabolism. Also you can concentrate better if you eat in the morning.

- A good start motivates one for the rest of the day.

Lunch

You will get nowhere if you start to run before you have learned how to walk. Start to change lunch and dinner only after you have gotten used to eating a good breakfast. Why do things the hard way? Eating those prepackaged cookies is a lot quicker than making a sandwich or a salad.

However, if you want to break the spell of binge eating, you will have to change your life style. Then you give up pre-packaged, pre-prepared food for delicious, nourishing and beneficial food. The question is not whether you can do this, but how you can integrate it slowly. You can look at this as a painful necessity, or you could welcome it with open arms. Your thoughts about this are the images that you yourself make of it. Next to eating away stress and binge eating attacks triggered by dieting, something else that impels you to overeat is seeing other people eating. If, for instance, you can't pass the bakery without buying all sorts of things and eating them, then it is better to stay away from places like that. Take your own lunch if you know deep inside that this works best for you, and take time to focus your attention on what you are eating.

The power of a warm meal

Ready-made food proportionally contains fewer nutrients, many calories and, above all, lots of artificial additives. We get considerably more energy from a fresh, unprocessed meal, which can be prepared in a short time. Pasta or rice, preferably whole grain, can be ready to serve within fifteen minutes. In the same time you can wok vegetables and, if necessary, add a salad and a vegetarian burger, fish or chicken. If you have more time, you can cook extra and put it in the freezer. If we learn to listen to the needs of our body, we eat hot soup when we are cold and not something like a cold salad with ice cream for dessert.

Moreover, a warm meal can be more satisfying, than something eaten cold.

Eating or drinking something warm sustains us when we are longing for emotional warmth in our life. There is a difference, however, between filling and feeding. I advise the person who has a tendency to feed herself chips, ice, licorice and fries, to try something different. By eating vegetables, fruit and whole grain products, you will discover eventually what is healthy and provides sufficient energy. If you want to avoid eating artificial additives, then choose organic food.

Priorities

Lisa: "I'm well-known for my ability to make everyone the most delicious meals, but I can't cook for myself. I don't like to eat alone. If I have to cook for myself, I don't seem to have the energy for it. And I can't think of a meal for myself."

Eating all the cookies in the jar, and that piece of chocolate, and a handful of cereal is going to play the leading part if we pay insufficient time and attention to ourselves. Maybe it's delicious, but we are missing essential building blocks (proteins and minerals) and will stay miserable. We don't want to feel like that, so there is the risk that we will start to eat a couple of snacks. If you are like Lisa, it is time for a change. It is a matter of planning, but it is possible. If even that little quarter of an hour to cook for ourselves doesn't fit into our schedule, it is time to seriously look at our life through a magnifying glass, because this is just a part of the problem: thinking everybody is worth the time, except you! If you put everyone else first, all that will be left for you will be the measly leftovers. It matters that we ourselves take responsibility for our lifestyle. Often, we have the tendency to blame everything else. There is always an excuse not to take sufficient time for breakfast, for exercise or to cook a healthy meal for ourselves. Not only is taking time to cook for yourself important, but also taking the time to eat your meal peacefully. Many people are completely unconscious of what they are eating because they are busy with other things. A way to maintain binge eating attacks is by not allowing yourself a moment's rest to eat. You can change this, for instance, by setting the table nicely, putting on relaxing music and taking time to sit at the table and eat peacefully. Don't let the phone disturb you, switch it off if necessary. Recently, I heard that a client, just after serving herself dinner, answered the phone. After finishing the conversation she saw that the food was gone, but she didn't have the feeling that she had eaten anything. Because of this sort of thing, you are not conscious of what you are eating, and you don't feel satisfied. You take the same risk by reading or watching TV when you are eating.[5] To develop a healthy eating-and-living pattern, you must change priorities, by putting yourself first. Take time to develop new and healthy eating habits and allow yourself to make mistakes with this. Every step in the right direction is worthwhile.

Exercise: eating mindfully

Sit at the table with the food in front of you. Relax, for instance, by taking a few deep breaths. You can thank the person who took the trouble to cook this meal. After that, pay attention to your food. Observe what it looks like and inhale the aromas. Try to eat slowly. There is less tendency to eat too much if we are conscious of what we are tasting. Chew well, so that your food becomes easier to digest. If you want to drink something, take a little sip, but don't rinse away your food with it. It takes some time before the sign that your stomach is full reaches your brain. You can slow down the tempo by putting your fork and knife down while chewing and picking them up after your mouth is empty. After dinner, take time to sit quietly for a little longer and feel how your body reacts to the meal.

Difficult moments

Every moment is a new chance.

Discover your real needs

Binge eating attacks can come on at the most inopportune moments, but often they are predictable. Unnoticed, it is possible we start to eat from force of habit. There are moments when we are used to eating something sweet. When we are used to eating something sweet while watching TV, we feel that need when we pick up the remote control. One client noticed that she always starts to eat candy when she is sitting in front of the TV. When she realized that, she decided to try something different, like playing the guitar or painting. Maybe you always take something to eat when reading or studying, or you eat sweets in the car. By eating at the table and not watching TV or reading at the same time, you disconnect activities that should not be connected with food.

I know former students who, when they open the refrigerator door, ask themselves: Am I really hungry? They close the door when they realize they are not really feeling hungry.

However, the person whose mind is preoccupied with food without signs of real hunger, should ask questions like: Do I have to eat this? Am I going to be happy because of this? What is my underlying need? Binge eating attacks often have a signal function. If our goal is to get rid of compulsive eating behavior quickly, then the chances are greater that we will fail.

Tamara: "I found out that I often had a binge eating attack when I did not give myself enough time to relax. I ate tensions away because I wanted to be liked by everyone and so I didn't dare to say no. Now, when I take time every day to consciously relax, it is a lot easier to say "no" to people when I don't feel like doing something."

On the road to healing, it is necessary to discover your true needs and to accept them. Tamara discovered that she started to eat when she needed to relax. Now she is capable of allowing herself, at a moment like that, to lie briefly on the couch and listen to beautiful music. At other moments a walk can relax her. However, we have to be conscious of the fact that we can't replace food by something as simple as a little walk, because when we don't really feel like doing that we don't satisfy our real need. Often, in the beginning, it is difficult to feed yourself in a different way. Food is easily accessible. It is available everywhere. It can be difficult to discover what your deeper need is, but as soon as you have discovered it, and it is no longer a secret, you will notice that food was actually a surrogate need; one that through habit and repetition developed a certain power over you.[6] Are you tired? Rest a little. Are you angry? Get it out in the open. Are you in need of warmth? Tell a loving person you need a hug. You won't succeed with this one day to the next, but if you pay attention more and more to your real needs, then you will eventually find, to your astonishment, that you have started to do other things than being preoccupied with food. It can happen unconsciously.

Vomiting, laxatives and diuretics

Elisabeth: "My mind tells me not to vomit, but when I have eaten too much I get a terrible stomach ache. Then it just has to get out. Otherwise I'm afraid I'll gain weight."

You can become addicted to vomiting, or using laxatives and diuretics. Often, it starts innocently, but before you know it there is another addiction. On top of that, the eating problem still exists and becomes even worse. Many diet pills are diuretics and can have nasty side effects. Those which work in a different way can be even more harmful. I have yet to discover the "wonder pill." Vomiting can come from habit, out of fear of gaining weight, or as a way of dealing with other fears and stress.

When women continue with binge eating, vomiting and the like, after a certain time they actually become fatter. Experience tells us, however, that our weight stays stable when we start to eat healthy.

Reasons to stop vomiting and the use of laxatives and diuretics:

- It becomes addictive, so you are stuck in a vicious circle.

- The more you vomit, the more your body will cry out for food, so you are going to eat more, vomit and so on. Because you only lose part of the food, you gain more weight anyway.

- Because of the vomiting, your salivary glands become swollen, so your face can look bloated. This can be the reason you think you have to lose more weight.

- Using laxatives and diuretics will not help you lose weight; the loss of fluid is only temporary. It is possible that because of this the body starts to produce hormones which cause you to retain fluid and start to feel heavier.

- Long-term use of laxatives leads to damage of the intestinal lining and to constipation. Because of that you need more and more laxatives.

- It leads to deficiencies in essential nutrients which can exacerbate the eating disorder.

- It can be very dangerous to your health (intestinal, kidney, liver and stomach problems, irregular heart beat, epileptic seizures and so on).

Tips for reducing vomiting, and intake of laxatives and diuretics:

- Examine your convictions about vomiting, laxatives and diuretics. Write them down and turn them into realistic thoughts.

- Write down, at a fixed time, what you hope to achieve in the coming week, regarding vomiting and the like. Keep the steps small in order to prevent disappointment!

- To get rid of vomiting, you can postpone it step by step. If you are vomiting right after you eat, you can start with postponing it for five minutes at a time. If you did this for a week, try in the next week to make the interval longer. If you had an extra binge eating attack, try your utmost to keep the food down.

- As long as you are still vomiting, brush your teeth after an hour, because the gastric juice is still present and will make your teeth vulnerable. You can rinse your mouth with water.

- Think about as many things as possible you could do right after dinner instead of vomiting. Put the accent on relaxing activities, where the chance is less likely that you will have negative thoughts. Monique does a puzzle after dinner, Sophia makes clothes and Natasha walks her dog.

- Slowly reduce your intake of laxatives and diuretics. It is possible that your body will retain the fluids when you suddenly stop taking these things. Take a little less every day, then cut back to every other day, every two days and so on.

- Keep in mind that you will suffer from constipation for a while. It is important to drink two quarts of water a day, eat healthy, especially vegetables and fruit, and to exercise daily.

- Two glasses of warm tea before breakfast can activate bowel movements. See for more suggestions chapter 6 (physical detoxification).

Every moment is a new chance

Recently, Beatrice vomited after she suffered a binge eating attack. She had the feeling she had failed and had to start all over again. But such an incident is no sign of weakness, it is a signal. She gave way to her feelings and observed tensions that she used to stifle with food. This was an opportunity for her to find the deeper meaning of this behavior. Thus, Beatrice began to understand how she could deal with it differently next time. Eating problems can re-emerge in times of stress. Tennis player Steffi Graf learned by patient practice to improve her relatively weak backhand and use it to attack, but when she was under high pressure she used to fall back on her old stroke. You can fall back on old habits when you are under pressure. But falling back is something completely different from sliding into total collapse. Don't punish yourself; that often leads only to new binge eating attacks. It is only human to land in an old trap now and then, but the choice is yours if you are going to get bogged down by low spirits. No matter how serious the situation is, you can always get out of it. Exercise is important for this.

There are more suggestions in appendix 1 which can help you in difficult times.

Be patient with yourself. A process of transformation goes together with falling and getting up again. Every moment is a new chance. You are searching for a balanced and fulfilling existence. Stop punishing yourself if it goes wrong; that can often lead to new binge eating attacks. You can use your energy better by thinking about what you want your life to look like.

Exercise: what am I really hungry for?

When we aren't physically hungry, we can ask ourselves at any difficult moment why we want to eat. You can do that with the help of the following questions:

1. What situation am I in? (Try to look at the situation as objectively as possible, without interpretation, comparison or labeling.)

2. What am I thinking? Challenge irrational thoughts immediately.

3. What do I feel?

4. What is my real need?

5. How can I fulfill this need?

6. How will I feel then?

7. What is going to be changed in a positive way in a year when I take my life in my own hands now?

If you don't have an answer to one question, move on to the next. It is possible that because of this, you will have an insight later into the previous question. If not, let go and try it some other time. You can write down the questions on a little card and put it in your appointment book or wallet.

Anita, for instance, wrote: "Wonder of wonders, this exercise helps me understand my real needs and give in to them."

1. *What situation am I in?*
   My boyfriend was coming over for dinner but something came up unexpectedly and he couldn't come.

2. *What am I thinking?*
   Although it is not his fault, I hate this. I looked forward so eagerly to our spending the evening together. Now that I am alone, I'm going to eat the whole dinner. What do I care, the day is ruined now anyway.

   Healthy thinker: I should not let this ruin my day. It is not going to make me more cheerful. I had intended to make it a relaxing and joyful day.

3. *What do I feel?*
   Loneliness and sorrow.

4. *What is my real need? What do I need?*
   I would like to have someone loving around me to talk to.

5. *How can I fill that need?*
   I'm going to call Kirsten and ask her out for tonight. If she is not available, I'll go to my sister. I always feel welcome there.

6. *How will I feel then?*
   I imagine that if I do that, I will feel more restful and powerful (and immediately I start to feel more restful).

7. *What will have changed in a positive way in a year if I take my life in my own hands now?*
   Then I will be radiant, healthy, energetic and powerful.

This exercise which is included in appendix 5 can be copied.

The different aspects of feeling hungry

If we know the difference between physical, psychological and spiritual hunger and learn to deal with that, our eating problem will be behind us.

Introduction

With compulsive eating behavior, we focus our needs primarily on the physical, most basic level. Although people will keep on eating, they will stay unfulfilled if deep inside they long for something else. The next summary shows the different aspects of hunger.

Physical hunger:
   Stomach hunger: a natural need of the body for food and fluid.
   Biochemical hunger: hunger that originates through a biochemical disturbance in the body.

Psychological hunger:
   Mental hunger: the need for knowledge and communication.
   Emotional hunger: the need for attention, togetherness, tenderness and intimacy.

Spiritual hunger:
   The longing to be who you truly are and the need to feel connected with a greater whole.

In this chapter, the focus is on physical and psychological hunger. The spiritual aspect of hunger runs through this book like a thread.

Physical hunger

Miranda said during the first day of training:

> "I made up my mind not to overeat anymore. I no longer have reasons to eat compulsively. I have a nice job, a dear boyfriend and lots of loving girlfriends. Through therapy I handled the unresolved problems from the past. How is it possible, then, that after a meal I don't feel satisfied and long for sweets? How is it possible that in this area I seem to have no will power?"

Stomach hunger exists through the need for food and food satisfies this need. The situation is different when there is a binge eating attack. We are feeling fine, there is no occasion to eat and suddenly there is this restlessness, this uncontrollable urge to eat, even though we have just had a meal. Women who have no eating problem recognize this when, for instance, they feel the urge to eat chocolate right before or during their period. I have written before that it is not a matter of will power. By regularly dieting and/or binge eating the body is knocked off balance. The connection between natural hunger and satisfaction is broken. So you can have a constant feeling of hunger even though you just had a large meal. You can be addicted mentally, as well as physically, to food. The boundary line is not easy to draw. They each have influence on each other. Psychological stress, for instance, raises our adrenaline and exhausts our energy reserves. Stress takes extra energy from the body in the form of glucose. That's why in stressful situations we have the tendency to look for food. If the body expects food, it will anticipate it automatically. When watching TV is coupled to food, your mouth will water as soon as you have the remote in your hands. Then the blood-sugar drops and that's why you experience an impulse to eat. This is the reason why you become, so to speak, physically addicted to food. Although you want nothing more than a balanced eating pattern, your body is accustomed to seductive stimuli and that's why it is often so difficult to break the spell of binge eating.

It can also happen that a biochemical disturbance can cause different eating behavior. A friend of mine, who is a physician, pointed out an extreme example to me. He told me that it is a well-known medical problem that people who have an iron deficiency sometimes suffer from a symptom called "pica," or in English, "strange urges." Another physician noticed that during meetings he was unthinkingly eating the plants. He had his blood checked and he indeed had an iron deficiency. Apparently deficiency diseases can lead to "strange urges."[7]

Factors that can cause biochemical hunger

Here is a list of factors that play a role in biochemical hunger:

Binge eating stimuli
- The body expects a binge eating attack.

Hereditary factors
- Physical: illnesses such as metabolic diseases, liver and adrenal problems.
- Psychological: depressions and the like.

Medicine
- Blood-pressure medication, corticosteroids and modern anti-psychotic medication.

Hormonal disturbances
- Thyroid gland and pancreas problems and Cushing's disease.

Neurotransmitters
- A low level of serotonin and endorphin (women are born with lower endorphin and serotonin levels than men).

Personal predisposition
- Especially sensitive people react (by means of a difference in biological vulnerability) very strongly to binge eating stimuli, addictive substances and artificial additives in food.

Stress
- Physical stress: gastrointestinal problems, food intolerance, fatigue.
- Psychological stress: negative thinking, pressure from work, problems in relationships, traumatic events.

Food
- Quick carbohydrates: sugar-free snacks, white bread, white rice, lemonade, alcohol.
- Caffeine: coffee, black tea, chocolate and cola.
- Too much saturated (animal) fat and too little polyunsaturated fats like fatty fish and avocado.
- Poor nutrition causes vitamin and mineral deficiency.
- Food intolerance.
- To yo-yo with food.

Illnesses
- Hereditary or acquired: brain damage and brain tumors.

However important physical factors are in compulsive eating behavior, we must still take into consideration our feelings and thoughts. During a lecture, I met a woman who suffered from bulimia and wondered if it had originated because she had too low a level of serotonin. Indeed, bulimia has been diagnosed in women with a low level of serotonin, so that they lack a feeling of satisfaction, but still that is not the only reason.

Our thoughts and emotions continually have an influence on our biochemistry. Factors that can lead to biochemical hunger form an extensive and complex matter about which much more will be known in the near future. A couple of factors have already been mentioned in this book. I will offer a limited explanation of food intolerance and the function of vitamins and minerals, with a couple of suggestions.

Food intolerance

The cause of food intolerance can be physical as well as psychological, or both.

When we don't express our anger, set our boundaries and repress natural longings, our body can protest by, for instance, developing intolerance to food. Sensitive people will reach this point sooner than others. When one habitually eats too much and eats food with too many additives, enzymes, and the metabolic, and immune systems go out of balance. This can lead to lack of energy, longing for sweets and all kinds of specific symptoms. The immune system can become so unsettled that it cannot fulfill its function of identifying certain nutrients and may perceive them as being strange to the body. Many apparent sources of food intolerance are: potatoes, chocolate, eggs, yeast, grains, coffee, peppers (bell peppers, red peppers etc.), dairy products, beef, oranges, sugar, wheat, tomatoes and pork. Food intolerance can lead to an eating problem. I know someone who is fully fixated on what she can't eat, and that's why she and her husband ended up socially isolated. The other way around it appears that someone is hiding behind food intolerance and saying: "I really can't help it if I can't eat certain products." You can stay in a vicious circle if you are addicted to food to which you have developed an intolerance. When we are eating as varied a diet as possible, the chance of developing a food intolerance is much smaller.

When someone reacts badly to certain foods, that does not mean that these should be avoided forever. If you discover which foods you cannot tolerate, you should avoid them for the present so that you stimulate the body as little as possible. But you can consider the psychological aspect, and with help, can work on healing of the organs and detoxification.

The function of vitamins and minerals

Vitamins and minerals are necessary for the body to function well. They strengthen the immune system, regulate the hormone system and fight fatigue. They make our nerves stronger, they improve concentration, help our skin stay beautiful longer and slow down the aging process. They form an important part of the enzyme system, regulate metabolism and are also responsible for biochemical reactions in the body.

Stress withdraws essential nutrients from the body. A deficiency in nutrients leads not only to physical symptoms, but also to psychological problems and can make people vulnerable to developing an eating disorder.

During the period that I suffered from bulimia and knew hardly anything about the importance of vitamins and minerals, I had a dream in which it was explained to me clearly that I had a calcium and magnesium deficiency. Also, this dream told me exactly which foods were rich in these minerals, among them tomatoes and bananas. Now, I am convinced that my eating disorder had caused me to develop a serious deficiency, so that I was trapped in a vicious cycle. Eating irregularly, choosing snacks and hardly any vegetables and fruit are all attacks on our health. Food today is polluted by pesticides and chemicals. Sugar and other refined foods deplete our bodies of vitamins and minerals. Smoking destroys vitamin C, and constricts and damages our arteries. The result is early aging that shows in the skin.

Alcohol depletes the body of fluid, folic acid and vitamin C, magnesium and calcium and is a burden on the liver. Caffeine is in products like chocolate, cola, coffee and black tea that, among other things, cause calcium and potassium depletion, which in turn, can lead to osteoporosis, palpitations and edema in the long run.

Here are a few examples of nutrient deficiencies. A deficiency of:

- chromium and zinc can lead to abnormal blood sugar levels and interfere with the burning of glucose.

- zinc, magnesium, selenium can interfere with the working of the pancreas and lead to eating disorders.

- manganese and selenium can interfere with the thyroid gland and with metabolism, which can lead to obesity.

- vitamin B3, folic acid, zinc and lithium can lead to depression and eating disorders.

- vitamin B5 causes, among other things, a low blood sugar level, dizziness and depression and can result in binge eating.

- vitamin B6 interferes with digestion of protein and leads to PMS.

A disturbed biochemical balance in your body can prevent you from taking a realistic look at yourself. For instance, you are slim, but you look at yourself as disgustingly fat. More little negative voices in your head are disturbing you, and you think you might as well be dead. My experience is that if you attack these problems on all levels, life (again) becomes worth living. You have to realize that food supplements are not a replacement for every day food, they are just that—supplements.

What to do?

Cindy: "For more than 25 years I suffered from binge eating attacks, which became worse and worse. Since I began to eat

regularly and a variety of healthy foods, I feel when I have
enough. If once I long for something sweet, then I eat it without
the old guilt. Sometimes I am surprised that I no longer have
the urge to start binge eating again. I feel energetic and cheerful. Most of my physical symptoms have disappeared. Also, I
am not afraid to go out on the streets. I've gotten over my fear
of driving and walking the dog."

Cindy's eating addiction of many years broke the connection
between natural hunger and fulfillment. She no longer knew how
it felt to give way to a natural need for food. Now she eats when
she feels hungry and she stops when she has had enough. She has
started to feel safe. Like everyone else, she encounters restlessness,
fear and problems, but now she can handle them effectively. In my
practice I see that many people very soon benefit from:

- eating highly nutritious and a variety of foods, omitting
  sugar-rich food in order to help the pancreas.

- using highly nutritious fats such as olive oil, safflower oil,
  linseed oil, in place of reduced fat, fat-free or deep fried
  fats.

- supplementing the vitamin and mineral deficiencies.

- exercising daily and relaxing.

Don't give up hope, but when you have biochemical symptoms
let an expert advise you. Keeping a temporary eating diary can give
you much insight, but with the help of an expert you will do better.
The cause of biochemical hunger is very complex. I prefer orthomolecular physicians or orthomolecular dieticians. These dieticians
work with vitamins, minerals and herbs, among other things.

The benefits of support like that are:

1. You are no longer alone in this, and therefore you will be more successful.

2. They know that when you have a biochemical disturbance you can have uncontrollable eating attacks and be fatigued.

3. They pay attention to the way in which the function of the pancreas, the liver and other involved organs can be improved.

4. They keep in mind your constitution (stature, body characteristics and metabolic type), specific symptoms and possible use of medication. Moreover, if, for instance, you have a disturbed intestinal flora, which makes it impossible for you to assimilate vitamin supplements or receive sufficient nourishment from food, that problem should be solved first.

5. You can also be treated with natural remedies for symptoms like anxiety, fear, depression, insomnia and the like. My experience is that the nervous system has to be brought to rest first, then the body normally follows. Advice is given about food, food supplements, plants and herb extracts.

Exercise: drinking water mindfully

Hunger can be confused with thirst. Do this experiment with water only. When you are thirsty, you can ask yourself: How do I know? What is the physical sign that lets me know? Where do I feel that? If I start to drink, how do I know when to stop? Which specific bodily sign is that?

This exercise is a good preparation for letting our body be our guide. In the same way, you can come to trust your ability to recognize the hunger for food. You can ask yourself the same questions with food as with water.

What we long for deep within

We are not unhappy because we have an eating problem, but we are having an eating problem because we are unhappy.

Psychological hunger

Psychological hunger can be mental as well as emotional. We get mental food from a good conversation, for instance, or from amassing knowledge, but here emotional hunger is the focal point. We can feed ourselves emotionally by discovering our emotional needs, recognizing them and, furthermore, talking about them. However, people with compulsive eating behavior do not have enough insight into their own emotions and needs, and so they don't profit from diets. Food is often used as emotional filling.

Inga called herself an "emotion-eater." She knew that she would keep on running to food unless she learned how to deal with problems in a different way.

Inga: "Now that I don't just fill up, but eat nourishing food, I don't feel hungry anymore, but I do have to deal with myself a lot. Because I was continually struggling with food, I lived more or less in a daze and I was only concerned about myself. Now that I no longer numb myself, I encounter things that I find very painful to face. Lately I had a quarrel with my boyfriend and after that conversation I automatically walked to the refrigerator. I opened it and suddenly realized that I wasn't feeling hungry, but that I wanted to eat away my frustration. I closed the refrigerator again, locked myself in my room, took my diary and wrote about it. Then I became calm again."

At the moment we are tempted the most to give in to our emotional hunger, our true self tries to change a part of our life. Feelings are to be experienced, not to be solved. Inga was used to "solving everything" with food. She was eating out of boredom and loneliness, because she missed something in her life to comfort herself in stressful situations. From the time Inga was young she was always willing to serve everyone around her. Like many women, she had never learned to ask herself what she wanted. Eating was as much her enemy as it was her best friend.

Through the training she found out what her feelings and needs were, and to comply with them in a nurturing manner. In that way, the longing for food was the beginning of a deep healing process.

On a regular basis I hear statements like: "If only I could get rid of my eating problem, then I will be happy." This is an illusion. Eating is misleading! If we focus specifically on that, then we don't see where the problem really lies.

If we are obsessed by food (to eat or not, what, where, counting calories, etc.) underlying problems entailing study, work, relationships, friends, family and so on, seem to disappear. This way of "dissolving" problems prevents us from dealing with them effectively. It also diverts us from pain, sorrow, fear or anger (from the past as well as now). Repressing such feelings only makes them worse. The real problems are not dealt with and as a result the eating obsession only increases.

Mara asked herself which inner emptiness she filled with food. I asked her: "Imagine that a good fairy appears to you and is capable of feeding you completely. She offers a magic spoon to you which holds precisely what you are really hungering for. What is it that she gives to you? It doesn't appear to be food, but loving attention." That was what Mara was longing for. That's how she discovered the true hunger that was the basis of her desire for food. Mara realized that for years she had been longing for a loving relationship and she "dissolved" that void by eating away her loneliness. When she discovered that to get loving attention she had to love herself first, the binge eating attacks disappeared. Our eating problem often offers, on a subconscious level, "the solution" by repressing our feelings and thoughts. When we learn to deal with this in a constructive way, our appetite will no longer be frightening. Then we are capable of separating physical hunger from psychological hunger.

Food as symbol

Like Mara, we can ask ourselves what food is telling us. When we stop to think about the food that we like to eat in such huge amounts we can discover what our choice of food has to say. We can connect certain foods with certain feelings and needs. For instance, we can use sweets as a surrogate for warmth, love, comfort and reward. When we always have the tendency to reach for sweets, do we really have enough experiences in our life which can be described as "sweet"? It can also mean that we have a tendency to keep ourselves "sweet." If you eat sugar-free products once in a while, do it on condition that you won't leave yourself out in the cold any longer, but will be nice to yourself. Then the pancreas can do its job. The longing for sugar however will decrease as you love yourself more, because then you are feeding yourself from within.

If we feel a need for salty, spicy food, it is possible that we need more zest in our lives. Crispy snacks are often associated with frustration or the need to express anger.

The examples given of the symbolic meaning of food are the general. I attach more value to the personal meaning that certain foods can have for someone. We can find out ourselves what our favorite binge eating food has to say to us. Our subconscious knows more than we are aware of and it can give us information through an internal dialogue.

Here are two examples:

Kiki: Creamy ice cream, why do I find you irresistible?

Ice cream: I am soft and sweet.

Kiki: That is precisely what I need in my life. I am sometimes too hard on myself. I set extremely high standards. I compensate for that by longing for sweetness and I give into that sometimes.

After a short break Kiki asks: How can I learn to open up to the soft, sweet side of myself?

Ice cream: I found that people can't resist me when I am melted.

Kiki (touched): Thank you; what you showed me is that underneath that hard-as-a-rock exterior is a soft side.

Laureen: Fudge, what is it that makes me think you are irresistible?

F: I am sweet and firm at the same time.

L: I can explain my need for something sweet, but what about the firmness?

F: You can't swallow me in one bite. First you have to chew a while on me, in contrast to most of the other food you eat.

L: Now that you mention it, indeed I'm used to swallowing my food at once, but I have to chew firmly on fudge for a while. Where does this need come from?

F: By sinking your teeth in this firmly you can get rid of aggression and built up stress in a natural way.

L: I wonder what makes me so aggressive?

F: You don't need to ask me, you already know the answer.

L: You're right, I would like to tell my partner and my mother what I think of them. I always try to keep peace, eating away all my frustrations for years, but now I am going to tell them what I really think of their behavior.

F: Very good, then you won't need me in large quantities any more!

Another technique is to make a drawing expressing your need for certain foods.

Emma: "On paper my need for chocolate suddenly became a big, brown bear. I felt protected by this strong bear, I could relax and I felt comforted. Never before had I realized my true needs."

Exercise: the symbolic meaning of your favorite food

Ask yourself what your favorite binge eating food stands for. What do you like about it? Which memories does it conjure up? What does it taste like? What pictures does it raise for you? Which feelings and longings does it bring to the surface? Carry on a dialogue as Kiki and Laureen did.

Don't reflect on it too much, then the answers will come by themselves.

You can also make a drawing and give expression with color and form to what a certain food means to you. Maybe you will find a symbol as Emma did.

Which feelings and needs bring that symbol to the surface?

5

A DIFFERENT LOOK AT YOUR BODY

The way we think about our body is the way we think about ourselves.

Liberating thoughts about your body

Positive thoughts strengthen your presence.

The pursuit of perfection

> Sabine: "You are disgustingly fat and ugly. You can't go out like that. I am going to send an excuse to my niece's wedding because you're a failure. Stop eating and go exercise."

Sabine's self-critic was talking again. She imagined that she looked terrible and she didn't dare show herself to the world looking like that. She had gained five pounds since the last family get-together. She panicked and, with a weak excuse, cancelled all her appointments. She made up her mind to show herself to the world again only when she reached her desired weight. Anyone who saw Sabine would not believe that this woman was insecure about her looks. She thought she was too fat, but this had nothing to do with reality. She struggled with imagined ugliness. What happens when we feel hurt, frustrated, insecure or threatened? Then it is "safer" to keep busy by dieting, reading or watching TV. Unfortunately, in the long run this is not the solution. When we suppress our feelings and the problems remain, irrational, negative thoughts multiply, and the eating problem gets worse. Once I read a saying that I'll never forget: "If you want to see what you were thinking yesterday, look at what your body looks like today. If you want to know what your body will look like tomorrow, look at what you are thinking today." The inner self and outward appearance are inextricably connected with each other.

What you think and feel inwardly you radiate outwardly. Habits that impede us, can be compared to downtrodden paths of our thinking, which are actually dead-end roads. There will be a change when we start to think realistically.

The desire to look beautiful as a cause?

Sabine hated herself because she hadn't succeeded in being perfect. Her self-esteem depended on how others judged her looks. It is not realistic to say that the way we look is not important. We all know that handsome and slender people are appreciated more in our society than ugly and fat people, but more things play a role in determining other peoples' appreciation. Feeling too fat does not always have to mean being too fat. I know heavy women who don't feel like they are too fat and slender women who feel they are fat. It is also possible that we feel fat one moment and slim the next, even when we can still wear the same clothes. My experience is that we can suddenly feel fat when we worry about something. The self-critic then predominates. It is often thought that the ideal of beauty should be blamed for an eating disorder like bulimia. In the advertising world, beauty and perfection are glorified. This can be a trigger, but it is not the cause.

There was for instance some research done among Iranian women. Some of them lived in the United States and they had a Western-orientated living-pattern; another group lived in Iran. The latter group was not influenced by Western culture and covered their bodies and heads. In contrast to their countrywomen in the United States, they didn't see slender models. Yet there were symptoms of eating disturbances among them; both groups demonstrated the same aversion to their own bodies.

This research proves that we have to put the problems in a wider context.

> Melissa: "It is that negative inner voice that has told me that I am not good enough as long as I can remember. This destructive image of myself has influenced my life negatively, in every way."

That negative voice can be compared with a broken record in our mind that constantly plays the same tune. What does this do to Melissa, to Sabine and to all the others if they hear that old, broken record day in and day out? They put on an act to those around them, they act as if everything is going smoothly, while they torment themselves daily with irrational thoughts.

We will hate ourselves more and more if we constantly bombard ourselves with negative thoughts.

Condemnation

Karen thought she was too fat and cut herself off from a boy she was in love with. She told me that she had first spoken to Ronald on the phone and that their contact was becoming more and more intense. She told him that " she wasn't the slimmest woman in the world," but he said that he didn't care. Now she had seen him once and she was completely confused.

It appeared from our conversation during this meeting that she constantly thought he must dislike her because she was too fat. I asked her to walk through the room in the same way she walked with Ronald. She immediately noticed that she was trying to make herself smaller. She said:" I hid myself." After that I asked her to walk through the room again, but now as her true self. And in one instant I saw a radiant Karen striding confidently. That same evening she called Ronald to make a new date. And now they have been living together for years.

Another example is Rose. I asked her to stand in front of the mirror and tell me what crossed her mind. She said: "My mind tells me that I look good, but deep inside I don't believe it." I asked her to tell me the negative convictions she had about her body. "I am a hideous, disgustingly fat and ugly human being." Rose had to make a choice: whether to continue suffering or to tell herself: enough is enough. I am fine just the way I am.

Miriam also condemned herself:

"As long as I can remember I have said to myself day after day: I am stupid and fat. I can't remember anyone else ever accusing me of that, but I think that since I was a little girl I have always believed it."

The seed of our later life lies in our youth. As long as she could remember, Miriam had thought of herself as not being good enough. Although she attended university and got good grades, she still believed she was not only fat, but also stupid. Now that she is thinking realistically, she can laugh about it.

We can judge ourselves, but the people around us can be ruthless, too. Clients tell me constantly that when they were children, their looks were criticized. If in the past your parents, brothers and sisters, gym teachers or friends told you that you had fat legs, or a funny nose or too-chubby cheeks, then it was automatically recorded on that tape in your head.

Tammy: "I still hear my father's voice telling me when I was twelve; 'Are you going out in those pants? I'm ashamed of you. Please put on different pants that hide your fat bottom.'"

Not the event, but what it means to us determines what our life will look like. A comment like that can be a contributing factor, but it is not the deepest cause of an eating problem. That cause lies in the meaning Tammy has given to it. It influenced the way in which she started to experience the world around her. I am certainly not saying it is her own fault. Nobody consciously chooses an eating problem.

It crept into our life and before we know it, it controls our life. We feel powerless if we don't know how to free ourselves from it, and we stay in that downward spiral. Although others have hurt us, we don't have to go on hurting ourselves.

It is not because of guilt that Tammy wanted to stop eating away her problems. It was the pain that she wanted to face and to deal with.

Challenging irrational thoughts about our body

By the time I first became conscious of the effect of negative convictions I had the following dream:

"I am in my parents house. I see the answering machine and want to listen to the messages. There are only old messages on the machine. I don't know how to erase them.

More and more often I realized that whenever I was thinking something ugly about myself again, this was in essence not me, but the saboteur in me. Through this insight I was able to distance myself from it, with compassion.

Which tape are you still listening to? What do you tell yourself day in and day out? What are the recurring thoughts when you look into the mirror? Imagine then that you take this tape out of the recorder and say to yourself: I will stop the negative words I say to myself. It is a new day. New thoughts belong to that."

Exercise: Challenging irrational thoughts about your body.

Draw a vertical line and write down on the left side all that pops up into your mind, the more the better.

Write the realistic thoughts on the right side. If you have problems turning irrational thoughts into rational thoughts, reread chapter 2.

An example by Miranda:

INNER SABOTEUR	RATIONAL THINKER
They don't like me because I am ugly and fat.	Nonsense, there are many people who want to be with me.
Would my partner still want me when I'm old, grey and full of wrinkles and have a fat, sagging body?	Okay, beauty is only skin deep, but if the way a person looks is very important to my partner, I can ask myself if that is a basis for a stable relationship.
Everybody has to think I'm beautiful.	Beauty is in the eye of the beholder; What is more important is that I accept my looks.
I gained 3 pounds	According to the weight charts I still have a normal weight.

Listening to your body

If I open up to the wisdom of my body,
then I know what I need.

Your body is the basis on which you live

"I hate my body," is a statement I often hear from my clients. They neglect or deny their bodies, misuse them or try to control them. But when we ignore signals from our body, we become estranged from ourselves. Then not only eating problems occur, but also physical problems, depression, auto-mutilation, fear, burn-out and problems with relationships. An example of auto-mutilation:

> Vera: "I don't know anymore how many times I pounded my head against the wall. At a certain moment I saw blood on the wallpaper and I realized that I had caused that. This brought me back to reality."

Our body is the basis on which we live, the starting point of our travel through life, but most people with an eating problem don't feel comfortable with their bodies. Vera became estranged from her own body. She wasn't in touch with it and she hated it. She had a picture of the "ideal body," and her own body did not match it. Later she expressed her feeling:

"I was not comfortable in my body, it disgusted me and I didn't dare to trust it at all. My breathing was often shallow. I was hardly aware of my legs. I was standing on them, walking with them and that was it."

If you compare the body with a house, fear drove Vera to the "attic." The reverse side of this is that bodily signals were not being noticed, or were being noticed too late, so Vera was hardly conscious of her feelings and needs. Our body is the connection between ourselves and the outside world. If we don't feel our body sufficiently, we keep on having problems with boundaries, for instance.

However, if we make connection with the richness of our body, we can express ourselves in a natural way and experience qualities such as love, power, surrender and clarity. It is important to literally and figuratively be down to earth with both feet on the ground. Then we are more capable of leading a self-assured and successful life. Vera learned to touch base with earth, that is, she made contact with the earth. If we do not really feel comfortable in our body and do not have both feet on the ground, then the energy will not flow sufficiently and we will soon be cold. We feel safer in a body that is warm, and with feet that are warm. When we are grounded, we can let go of stress more easily.

Exercise: the tree

Stand upright, feet no wider apart then the width of your hips, toes a little inwards, your knees bent a little. Close your eyes. See yourself as a very powerful tree, which has roots that reach deep into the earth. Feel how your feet are connected with the earth and take in the energy of the earth. Imagine that through your roots you are being fed by the earth. Let whatever stress there may be disappear into the earth through the roots. This tree's roots are connected with the earth and its branches reach to the sky. The sap in the innermost core flows from top to bottom and from bottom to top like a long, deep and peaceful breath.

After approximately five minutes, open your eyes again. Stretch and move around a bit.

The power of mind-body therapy

Nina said on first acquaintance:

> "Because of therapeutic conversations I have had in the past, I understand how things are, but it doesn't solve my eating problem."

Our body expresses the story of our life. Each thought, and each sensation, has a direct effect on our body and vice versa. Our posture reflects how we are feeling. The processing of emotions by our body happens sometimes consciously, but mostly unconsciously. When emotional problems last a long time, it means that emotions are being repressed and needs are being neglected, and that affects our bodies in the shape of physical symptoms. The consciousness training works with mind-body therapy. This method not only purifies the body, it relaxes and vitalizes it. Our body is always present in the here and now. The goal is to familiarize yourself with your body and to learn to listen to the signals that it gives. You learn how you can be in contact with your body in a relaxed way. By being aware of the signals given by your body and understanding their meaning, you can find out who you are and what is important to you. It is a way to make direct contact with your feelings. Our body reflects how we deal with feelings like pain, fear and longing. This way we come into contact with destructive core convictions like "I am not good enough," "I weigh too much," or "I am not worthy to be loved." Through mind-body therapy we learn to know ourselves beyond the rational.

Physical pain as a signal function

Among indigenous peoples it is normal to listen to the signals of
the body, but in Western culture, alas, it is different. Our body is
the purest measure; it constantly gives signals of anything that is
out of balance, but most people have not learned to listen to it. An
example is provided by Helen, whose stomach spoke clearly. For
days she had stomach pain. Luckily, she habitually consulted her
GP when she had a new or unusual symptom, but now there was
no particular diagnosis. During the session we discussed what this
powerful signal meant. I invited her to close her eyes and to imagine that her stomach had a voice. The voice said: "I am dark, cold
and oppressed and my need is rest and relaxation."

Her stomach told her in clear language how she could take care
of it, and she promised her stomach she would listen to it. In the
end, she thanked her stomach. In time, after this inner dialogue,
her stomach pain disappeared.

Gisela was referred by her GP. She often visited him with severe
intestinal problems. She was examined thoroughly by a specialist,
who could not find anything wrong. For a couple of years she also
consulted a dietician, but still she had symptoms. When for the
hundredth time she went to see her GP because of her abdominal
problems, she confessed that she had not really managed to deal
with food and thought that maybe she should try working on that.
After participating for a month in the training, her intestinal problems completely disappeared.

Another example is Renée. She was asked to fulfill a manage-
ment position with more responsibility. Her mind said, "You can
handle this position," but her whole body protested. After this offer
was made to her, she suffered from shortness of breath, palpitations
and stiff shoulders.

Now that she was no longer eating away the stress, she felt
much stronger and knew that deep in her heart she didn't want
this responsibility. After two days she said "No." She felt relieved
immediately and her symptoms disappeared.

Renée achieved clarity by listening to the signals of her body and by being honest. She wrote:

> "Now that my eating behavior has started to normalize, I notice that my feelings are coming more and more to the surface. I notice little bodily signals and I listen to them. The beauty of it is that not for a moment do I lose control, I just let it come."

Finally, there is the story of Linda, who had to exercise for at least three hours a day. Her 'inner saboteur' forced her to do that, while her skinny body almost collapsed. At the age of fifteen, she had already been diagnosed with degenerated cartilage. During a relaxation exercise when she was lying on a mattress, she confessed softly that she was tired and wanted more than anything to lie down. Linda is learning more and more to listen to her bodily signals. If she is feeling fatigued, she dares to admit it. Compulsive exercising belongs to the past. She no longer demands perfection from herself.

Linda now realizes that to learn to listen to her bodily signals doesn't lead to loss of control, but, that on the contrary, you become more and more the master of your existence. Her body was a hated opponent, but has now become a companion.

Exercise: letter to your body

Write a letter to your body. Here is an example.

Dear Body,

    I've known you since you were born, but I lost you for a while. I didn't appreciate you, even hated you and thought you were a hindrance. I looked at you only as equipment for moving and as a necessary manifestation

for other people, but not as something I could enjoy. If I
did not feel safe, I broke contact with you by fantasizing
that I did not feel the pain and restlessness in you. Now
I can finally see who you really are: a wondrous body
that gives me uncountable possibilities. I neglected you
for a long time, though you were faithful and kept on
functioning. I can see now that you never deserved to be
neglected, that you should be pampered and cherished
instead, because you are fine just the way you are and
because you belong to me. I won't leave you again.

Love,
Fiona

Be prepared to get a letter back.

Dear Fiona,

I am glad that we have contact again. We are insepa-
rable. There is nothing that I want more than that you
should be well. I am not against you, I just want to be
there for you; after all, we are one. We are in this together
again.

Love,
You know who.

Sexuality

In sexuality we can encounter ourselves to the maximum.

Introduction

> Monique: "Although he says I have a beautiful body, I don't
> believe him. I only dare to give myself to him when I have been
> drinking. I prefer to make love under the sheets in the dark. As
> soon as he touches me I feel confronted with my body and all
> kinds of negative thoughts run through my mind. I hold in my
> stomach and try to lie in the most flattering position possible."

It seems that people most identify themselves with their bodies.
Naturally, being insecure plays an important role in relationships.
There are women who, because of that, don't dare to start a relationship. Often, I overhear new clients who have a partner saying that
their love life is not booming. The tendency to control everything
does not lead to a satisfying love life. When we have insufficient
contact with our body, sexuality can be a threat. We can think that
we have to stay in control or we are afraid to give ourselves up to
something that is unknown. Maybe we believe that our longing is
too strong and that it will never be lived up to. We are not capable
of getting in touch with the kinds of feelings and needs that are
present in our body, let alone making connection with and enjoy-

ing the other. We will only be full of life when we are fully present in the here and now and connect ourselves with our body and our passion. There can only be actual surrender if we can let go of judgments and expectations about ourselves and the other. Openness, vulnerability and willingness to give as well as to receive are essential to this. The distance between partners fades when they dare to be vulnerable. We are all vulnerable creatures. Recognizing our vulnerable side is the road to self-knowledge and acceptance of ourselves. Power lies in being conscious of our vulnerability. I learned this during a week of training that a colleague and I taught about sexuality. After a certain time, the participants each dared to be vulnerable and because of that, radiated enormous strength.

Nowadays, people seem to be very open about sexuality, but often that is pretence. Unfortunately, this is still a very sensitive area. Many hardly dare to admit that they find it hard to talk about. The first step would have been taken if they would talk about it.

Convictions regarding sexuality

Amelia: "I often heard my oldest sister say: 'Sweetie, the first time hurts so much,' and her face spoke volumes. As soon as a boy made advances to me in any way, I couldn't get away quickly enough. The first time I made love to a boy I was so tense that I wanted to stop, but there was also a little voice inside me that said I would then be over with it. (The first time would be painful no matter what). Years later I heard stories from girlfriends and I realized that a first experience can be nice, too."

Convictions regarding sexuality can leave behind deep traces. Gabi is another example. Her father also brought a message that raised fear.

Gabi: "When boys started to pay special attention to me, my father took me aside. He said in a serious voice without further explanation: 'Nobody is allowed to touch you.' This had a lot of impact for a long time. As soon as a man came close to me and started to make advances, I heard, so to speak, the voice of my father. I felt fear and froze on the spot."

The message that Gabi got was: Men mean danger! Now that she is as an adult and is aware of that, she says: "I've replaced this old, destructive message with a new, realistic conviction."

Mandy: "What man would want me? I don't have anything to offer and I'm not good looking, so I am unattractive to men."

Mandy found out that she radiated what she believed. Sexual attractiveness goes beyond your looks.

In the last part of this chapter I will go more deeply into this. One thing is for sure: if you start to find yourself attractive, you will radiate that to others.

Sex out of a longing for love

Fini: "I alternated binge eating attacks with periods of hardly eating anything. I have to work out something with men. In addition to my boyfriend, for years I have had a lover. Lately, I had a little adventurous fling with a third man. When that happened I thought: this, I believe, is wrong. Not only am I addicted to food, but also to men. It is time that I thoroughly investigate my addiction pattern."

Fini liked the temporary attention of men, but that didn't bring her what she was searching for deep inside.

Just as with her binge eating attacks, she started to see the long-run damaging consequences. Men can be used as a quick "shot," just like an eating binge. Sex can be a means of experiencing that little spark of intimacy for a while. When we don't know how to take care of ourselves, in the area of eating as well as in association with others, there is the risk that we will attract the wrong partners. If you hide your feelings with food and have no respect for yourself, how can you expect others to respect you?

After binge eating you can still feel empty, just as with "bad" partners. If you think that fulfillment is outside yourself, you will remain unfulfilled and unhappy. If we start with the idea that we will find success in work or money from food, alcohol, or love, we will never fill our inner emptiness. It is never enough!

When you are young and have a healthy attitude, you can go through a phase in which you feel the need to experiment with sex and a lot of brief relationships. When it is a pattern that you get bored easily and move on and on to the next "prince," stop and think about what you are really longing for.

> Sarah: "I started to recognize the inward struggle between my limited self and my true self. My limited self wanted to gorge, to drink or have sex with the first man who paid a little attention to me. But now that I am in touch with my true self, I can feel what I really need."

At first, Sarah chose temporary pleasure, but now she knows what she is longing for deep inside, and so she has the strength to resist the "temptation" and be faithful to what she most desires: accepting herself. That doesn't mean that she is no longer open to the natural longing for union with a partner. The need to be united, to transform sexual energy into all-embracing love, is a basic longing. However, we will only bond freely with a partner if we first take responsibility for our own happiness.

Sexual abuse

Setting boundaries is the ability to differentiate between your own feelings and responsibilities and those of others. Boundaries bring a feeling of safety. The safer you feel, the more you can be yourself. It is possible that, at a young age, boundaries were not set, or not respected, for example, in the case of sexual abuse.

One who experienced this in youth, is influenced by it later in life. There are people who believe that it was their fault. Although the abuse might have stopped, the feeling of shame can persist and be carried throughout one's life.

For example, Stephanie was ashamed because when she was seven years old she "let it happen." She thought: I must have encouraged it, so maybe I could have prevented it. She blamed herself for something she could not control. In addition, it is often someone you love and are dependent on. That makes the situation even more confusing; boundaries are not respected and the reaction to this can be disturbed eating behavior. Normally, sexuality is something you grow into. When one is confronted with sexual abuse as a child, one is affected in the crudest way.

Janie found a "solution" to dealing with this.

> Janie: "When I was 12 years old, I was suddenly molested from behind on the street. From that moment on I decided subconsciously that if I became fat I would be less attractive prey to men. I realized that only after I read a book which deals with the subject."

This incident is to be compared with a burn. It happens in an instant, but the scar remains. You can be mentally, as well as physically, scarred. You burn yourself just for a moment, but the aftermath is for life. The abuse can last a day, a month or a year, but the consequences will go on until you decide to do something about it.

When I met Janie she was really overweight. Her eating problem was endangering her health. The price she paid was too high.

During training, she realized that as a young girl she had developed a survival strategy, but now that she was a grown woman, she no longer needed this layer of fat to protect her, which she had carried around for over 20 years. Mostly it is not the traumas that make us emotionally ill, but the inability to bring them out in the open. Subconsciously, we think that we can't deal with it, and as a child that was true, but as an adult maybe we can take another shot at it.

With help, respect, and by taking small steps, Janie could look the fear from the past in the eye and leave it behind. The binge eating attacks have disappeared. Through follow-ups, I keep in touch with her. For the first time, she has a relationship that has lasted for a year and recently I received a little card announcing that they are going to move into together.

Exercise: letting love in

Sit in a comfortable position and concentrate on your breathing without trying to influence it. Think about a situation in which you felt love. Take a deep breath and let this love flow deep inside without associating it with a certain person, a pet or particular situation. If you allow this love to flow through you in this way, your body will respond positively.

Acceptance

I have a body, but I am infinitely more than that.

How long will you let your life be controlled by the self-critic?

The person who looks at herself in the mirror and says: "I look beautiful," is quickly going to be labeled as vain and arrogant. If we receive a compliment on our looks, many women start to tone it down; women are capable of cutting themselves down and trying to look as good as possible at the same time, because then you will be approached in a more positive way. Who can resist this double morality?

We can't attach our happiness to having a perfect nose or the right cup size. In a woman's magazine I once read a story about a woman who had her first cosmetic surgery done fifteen years earlier. Since then she has had many more, because there was always something that she thought was not perfect. A couple of years ago a poster hung in the window of the Bodyshop with the following text: "There are three billion women who don't look like a super model and only eight who do." Accepting our body starts with skipping comparisons and learning to look at ourselves without condemnation. To many a woman, self-image and happiness depend on reaching her goal weight, but the euphoria is mostly temporary. Discontent with our body is synonymous with discontent with ourselves.

Most people can't accept themselves the way they are; they want to be perfect and to look perfect. It is the voice of the self-critic which is never satisfied, who only sees what is "wrong" and constantly says: "You are not good enough."

Making peace

Sonya, an old acquaintance of mine, struggled with her figure almost her whole life. She is reaching menopause now, which is causing her body to change, but she refuses to accept that. So, day in and day out, she is busy exercising and dieting in order to fit into her old clothes again. Although her figure is beautiful in the eyes of everyone who knows her, she herself will never agree with them on this.

Where Sonya chooses to suffer, Jessica now has buried the hatchet.

> Jessica: "Although I got compliments on my figure, I always felt fat. I starved myself, but my round hips remained. I know now that there are different types of bodies. Round, straight, pyramid-shape or upside-down pyramid. The accent is always on one of the four. I have the classical female round build. Now that I have accepted this, I am at peace. I will never get the straight build I see on others and I don't long for that anymore. I am satisfied with my body and my firm thighs. That is also me! Sometimes my thighs are suddenly in the way. Now I know that when there is something else I worry about, they serve as a signal, just as binge eating served as a signal in the past."

For as long as she could remember, Jessica had problems dealing with her body. She thought that her thighs were too fat and her breasts too big. She also thought that her stomach and bottom were too round. It took her years to find out that severe dieting, promptly followed by binge eating, was not the solution: she kept her "roundness" because that was the way she was built.

Frederique presents another example of a positive body-experience.

> Frederique: "During a visualization, I was asked to imagine my ideal figure. To my own astonishment, I found that I didn't want to be skinny. It seemed that I already had my ideal figure. Finally, I had accepted it and I could say to myself, 'My body is fine just the way it is!'"

Often, clients want to have a normal life, but they don't want to change their behavior. They hold on to a "false safety net." Petra said that she wanted to have slimmer legs before she stopped vomiting and using laxatives. To cease that kind of behavior would mean letting go of what is reliable and familiar, and letting go can be frightening. Each choice requires a sacrifice. As long as there is a "but," we are not prepared to look the truth in the eye. If we really want to get rid of our binge eating, we have to find out what this "but" stands for.

Recently, I met an acquaintance whom I had not seen for quite a while. She told me at great length why she was fatter than before. I didn't even notice that; to me she is a woman who radiates warmth. I love her as she is. Unfortunately, a big size is condemned in our society. From there it is a small step to condemning ourselves. When we accept our bodies, we experience less stress and will have less tendency to eat when we are not hungry. Feeling fat leads quickly to a feeling of guilt, shame and self-punishment. That can end in binge eating, which makes us feel fatter and which can lead to severe dieting or even fasting. When we neglect or misuse our body, it will leave us in the lurch. This will change only if we treat our body with respect.

> Hannah: "I bought body lotion and as I was putting it on, for the first time in years, I stood naked in front of the mirror. After I was done with the lotion I worked up the courage to

look at myself from all sides. I have been doing this now for two weeks and I notice that I'm starting to like this ritual. While I'm putting on the lotion I pay extra attention to my stomach. That part of me is starting to belong to me more and more."

Since puberty, Hannah had suffered from binge eating and she was heavily over-weight when she started the training. She hated her stomach the most. She told me that she always automatically covered it with her hands. As a result of an individual session she said that she no longer wanted to neglect her body, but wanted to begin to pay conscious attention to it. She started to exercise more and in connection with the plan of steps to take (see Chapter 2: Strike a Balance) she thought of putting on body lotion after taking a shower.

If we are paying loving attention to our body we can listen better to the signals it gives us. This makes it easier to recognize the difference between physical and emotional hunger. When you have a balanced living-pattern, the natural balance of your body can repair itself.

A remark that I want to make here is that size 8 is not for everyone. That is a struggle that most women will lose. Strike out the words "ideal-weight" forever from your vocabulary. Don't wait to start living until the scale gives you permission.

We can trust our body to be wise, it knows exactly which weight suits us. This is subject to change: menstruation, pregnancy, breastfeeding and, last but not least, menopause influence it. Nora, a client whom I now see only once in a while for a follow-up, said recently:

"I left the illusion behind that I have to have a perfect body. I have learned to accept it as it is, with my beautiful and less beautiful sides. That also means that I have to make peace with getting older. That I get more and more wrinkles and gray hair is no longer strange to me. Rise, shine and fade away, that is the reality. My self-esteem no longer depends on how I look. It is grounded now in deeper values."

Sometimes, I overhear menopausal women say that they dream they are having a baby. This can mean a new phase in life, a rebirth. What I noticed with Nora, and also with other women who deal with this phase in a natural way, is that they aren't bothered so much anymore. They no longer have to prove themselves. They have become calmer and wiser. If we derive our identity from beauty and slenderness, then we are going to have more problems when we get older. We can't stop the fact that our body is changing in a natural way. We can be obsessed by this, or focus on more important things. If we fight against it, it will hurt, but if we accept that natural process, then we will profit from it.

A saying that is a source of inspiration for me as for many others is, "God (or another higher power) give me the strength to accept the things that I can't change, the courage to change the things I can change and the wisdom to know the difference."

Power of attraction

We all have seen someone who looks attractive, but lacks radiance. One's inner self and outward appearance are inextricably connected with each other.

Being beautiful or pretty is something that is genetically determined, but it does not necessarily coincide with an attractive radiance. True beauty comes from within.

This is connected with self-confidence, self-esteem and allowing ourselves to enjoy. Attraction goes beyond the shape of your face, the length of your legs or the size of your waist. An attractive person has radiance and that is something everybody can develop.

You can choose to be a radiant, attractive personality. You are as attractive as you think you are. I know many women who, regardless of their age or appearance, have no trouble attracting positive attention. They radiate charisma. They think of themselves as worthwhile and the possessor of a captivating personality. A magnetic power of attraction coincides with certain qualities.

People are beautiful by, for instance, the power, compassion and wisdom that they radiate. Others look at you in the same way that you look at yourself. The times that I have heard someone say that she was ugly and fat are countless. What kind of message does this send to those around you? Precisely, others will see you in the same way.

An example is provided by Wilma. She thought it was normal to spend time and money on her family, but not on herself. She didn't even buy a pair of earrings, because she said literally, "I'm not worth it." She expressed indignation that she was used as a doormat by her husband and children, but she didn't see that she was sending them a message that she didn't matter. Not a positive example to pass on to your children. Now that she thinks of herself as a valuable woman, she says:

> "I didn't think I was worth spending money on, but now I don't only invest in who I am, but also in how I look. Sometimes, to my astonishment, I still notice that my family reacts positively to this."

Investing in your looks can do a lot, but the most important requirement to being attractive is believing that you are attractive. Feeding your mind consciously with positive thoughts has a unprecedented effect on your radiance and with that you can bring about big changes in a very short time. You can feel as radiant as anyone else and the more you become convinced of it, the more those around will take notice of that.

Carol: "In the past I wanted to have everything under control in order to get through the day. I felt insecure because I wanted to look perfect and slender, but I never looked like that in my own eyes. With this uptight attitude I didn't, of course, emit the radiance I wanted to. I feel relaxed now and much more attractive. Even though I gain weight and people comment on that, it doesn't upset me anymore. I am worthwhile."

It will strike you that the more your self-confidence grows and the more attractive you become, the less occupied you are by how you look. Carol, who suffered from bulimia for years, now has a natural brilliance—she is herself.

Exercise: cherishing yourself

Imagine that you are smiling lovingly at a baby. In the same loving way you can smile at yourself. Start first with your organs: your heart, your lungs, your kidneys, and so on. When you feel confident with that, you can smile at your feet, your shins and then slowly up to your head. Linger a little longer at the parts of your body that could use some extra love.

6

CLEAN UP

———

Cleaning up is letting go.

Physical detoxification

Taking care of your car and not taking care of yourself?

Introduction

We have, literally and figuratively, a bone to pick with life. That applies as much to food as to life-experiences.

When we are capable of digesting what we "have on our plate," we won't have to carry around the undigested leftovers. The snake is a symbol of healing and represents change and renewal. On a regular basis it sheds its skin and that is a symbol of death and rebirth. We, too, can feel ourselves reborn when we let go of our "old skin." Most clients who have just started the training exhibit, along with psychological problems, many chronic physical symptoms such as headaches, digestive difficulties, skin problems, joint aches, concentration problems and fatigue. The body and mind influence each other. If you attack problems in the psychological as well as in the physical area, you will break through the vicious cycle more quickly.

Detoxification

The oldest medical method of treatment, ayurveda, I look upon as an important source of inspiration. Once I read an interview with an ayurvedic physician who said that Westerners have so many chronic symptoms because they don't detoxify on a regular basis. The idea that chronic illnesses can result from the poisoning of the metabolism has become more accepted over the last couple of years. Harmful substances which are ingested via food and water or inhaled from polluted air can lead to an accumulation of poisons in the body, especially in the intestines. The nervous system, the gastrointestinal tract, the hormone and immune systems are much influenced by that, but the organ that suffers the most from these poisons is the liver. This "waste-disposal service" has to deal with three streams of poison on a daily basis:

- external poison (the above-mentioned harmful substances)

- internal poison (by not sufficiently digesting, parasites and the like)

- emotional poison (like negative thoughts, jealousy, depression, emotions that have not been dealt with).

The liver is the most important organ that controls the blood sugar level. Liver processes are influenced by substances with a regulating role function (like hormones) from other organs. The liver is important if the body is to function well. Disturbances of the liver not only influence the functioning of the other organs and tissue, but also the metabolism, blood quality and quantity, immune function, hormone regulation, vitality and our psyche. A dysfunctional liver causes depression. Harmful substances exist in the body often as the result of unbalanced intestinal flora, especially the skin, the lungs and the intestinal mucosa react to this. If the body is not capable of getting rid of all those substances, they can literally come out through the skin.

Nancy: "For years I had physical symptoms, but I was used to it so I paid no attention to them. My face was one of the few parts of my body that I was content with. To my horror, I got a skin disorder just there. I felt very insecure because of that. It was as if my mask had fallen off and now everyone could read on my face that I was not doing well. Now that I live more consciously and lead a healthy life I feel better in every way. You can see it on my skin."

The more Nancy chose a healthy lifestyle, the easier it was to let go of what was polluting her body. Not only can our body show us that it is polluted, but our dreams can tell us that too. A friend of mine had three dreams about "pollution" within a short period of time. The first dream was about a washing machine that broke down. The second dream was about his bathroom that, to the dreamer's astonishment, was very dirty. In the last dream, the kitchen needed to be painted. A year ago, he had installed a new kitchen and a new bathroom. This dream was trying to tell him something else. He knew that his body was also his dwelling, but he wanted to make sure so he had himself examined by a physician. His dreams had warned him correctly. His liver was heavily contaminated and needed thorough cleansing.

If we want to restore the metabolic balance, the toxic stream supply has to be cut off as much as possible and its discharge has to be supported. The production of internal toxins can be reduced by eating food which contain no harmful ingredients and by improving the digestion. This can be done by, for instance, normalizing the production of gastric juices and balancing the intestinal flora. This will result in better digestion and an increased absorption of nutrients. Chronic digestive disorders can be treated well with phyto-therapy, in the form of plant and herb extracts. In France, Germany and Switzerland this is an important part of official medical science. They have had experience with this for centuries, and, in the last fifty years, the literature in this scientific area has grown enormously. If we can acknowledge that the liver has reached its limits regarding processing toxins, then we can understand the increasing need for safe medications. There are many of these medications on the market for you to try out yourself, but considering the complexity of eating problems, self-medication is not advisable. Consult with an orthomolecular physician, a nature physician or an orthomolecular dietician. They use, among other things, phytotherapy.

Simple ways for detoxification

- *Purification cleansing*

  One of the cheapest ways to cleanse our body of waste materials is the ginger-tea cure, originated by the ayurveda. This raises your concentration, improves the circulation and digestion, lessens the need for sweets and increases your vitality! This purification cleansing, which lasts six weeks, can be done at the start of every season. You will find the recipe below.

  In the morning, boil about 2.5 pints mineral water or purified water. After twenty minutes, pour the rest of the boiled water in a thermos flask. Add a piece of ginger root (0.5 to 1 inch, as needed). During the day, drink little sips of the hot water from the thermos flask; if the ginger becomes too dominant you can add more water. The water has to be as hot as you can drink it without burning your tongue. Each time, drink enough to give you a pleasant feeling in your stomach. If you don't feel like taking a sip, don't force it. If the water is too hot for you, let it cool off a bit. This tea will help to get rid of the waste materials through the intestines, kidneys and skin. The hot water works more powerfully than two pints of purified water unheated. At the same time, both the digestion and the metabolic energy improve. For those who can't tolerate ginger , turmeric is an alternative.

  In the beginning, itchiness, hot flashes, nausea or congestion may occur. That means that waste materials are being released. If you suffer from these reactions, let the water cool a little more before drinking it.

- *Drinking enough water*
  In the morning keep a big bottle of purified water on hand (see purifying cure above). When this is empty by the evening you know you will have drunk at least 1 pint of water. When you are on the road, it's a good idea to always have water with you. Feelings of hunger are often confused with thirst, so, when in doubt, drink a large glass of water before eating. Do that, too, when you are fatigued. Normally after five minutes you will notice the difference.

- *Exercise daily* (see chapter 3: Energy gluttons and Energy Givers).

- *Healthy food* (see chapter 4 Back to Basics).

- *Visualization*
  In addition to different exercises from this book, you can do the following. My friend twice dreamt that his house needed cleaning. Imagine that your house needs cleaning. Feel what it needs. Clear away everything that is unnecessary. You can do this literally, too! Finally, one more marginal note: a fasting cure is also a detoxification method, but I don't advise people with compulsive eating problems to fast, because experience has shown that, after that, they tend to revert to extreme eating behavior.

Exercise: stomach massage

This simple massage technique originates from qi gong. You stimulate the small intestine as well as the colon. It improves the digestion and excretion and increases energy. You can stand up (bend the knees a little), sit or lie down. Put your right hand on your navel and your left hand on your right hand (men vice versa). Make light, circular movements to the left across your stomach. Start small, make the circles bigger and bigger, while your hands stay on your navel. After a while make the circles smaller again. Let your hands rest on the navel for a moment. Than make the same movements in the other direction. Do this as well to the left as to the right for about 5 minutes. Rest comfortably for a while.

Emotional detoxification

The key to really opening up is not thinking, but feeling.

Dealing with feelings

Soon after Vivian ended her relationship, she had the following dream:

> "I am going to throw a huge party, but first I am going to clean the floor. I vacuum, but that doesn't seem to be enough. There are stains on the linoleum, which I have to get out. I receive a scouring pad from someone I don't know and with this 'correct' tool, the stains are easily removed. The party can begin."

The relationship with this partner had left tracks. Before the party could start, this client had to clean up. Vivian wanted to erase feelings like pain, sorrow, anger and fear. Everyone longs for wholeness, but we won't experience that as long as we are running away from painful feelings. They secure themselves in our body if we repress them, with everything that goes with it. Pain is inevitable, but if we empty our backpack, the bottom seems to be covered with little pearls which we only have to pick up. Under the pain and the awareness of it, lies a deeper insight, and freedom. If we want to leave compulsive eating behind, it is absolutely necessary that we deal with emotions in a different way. If we learn to cope with small irritations, we will have less tendency to eat them away. Thus we prevent things from piling up. Moreover, the better we deal with small every day problems the better we deal with big ones.

> Zoë: "Nowadays I deal with everyday irritation in this way. First, I give the irritation a score from 1 to 10. Then I imagine a pink balloon and I put that irritation inside it. I pick up the balloon and take a deep breath. I relax my hand, letting go of the balloon and breathing out at the same time. I repeat this until the emotion is reduced to zero."

What Zoë describes is useful in many situations, not only with upsetting emotions, but also with joyful, euphoric ones. When emotions throw us off balance, we might start binge eating. The person with high expectations can well be disappointed. If you are, for instance, extremely happy that a precious friend is stopping by, there is the risk that you will be disappointed. However, if you are open-minded, you are capable of being in the here and now, and of enjoying what the moment brings.

From depression to expression

> Arianne: "I was very depressed, deeply fearful and was incapable of working. Through consciousness training I discovered how I could change depression into expression. This helped to release my creative stream. I now get fulfillment from painting."

During the training, we work with different ways to express feelings. Next to psychotherapy and body-focused therapy, we work with creative forms of expression like role play, dance and movement expression, creative writing, voice expression, drawing and painting. Creative expression connects us with our feelings.

We can heal by starting to move things; literally moving by danc-ing, the life-energy streaming through our bodies, or expressing what lives in us by drawing. One person may benefit from using her voice, another by writing poems or by dancing her own dance. One form is not better than another. The challenge is to find out what best suits you. Often, clients are tormented by the inner critic that tells them that their method of expression has to be perfect. But perfection doesn't offer room for change, while, on the other hand, life is a synonym for change.

We can't do this right or wrong, we can only do it. If you want to take on the challenge, start small, so that there is more chance that you will enjoy it. It is impossible to go into all the forms of expression in this book. One example is drawing or painting the inner critic. In this way, we learn another language. Once the critic is on paper he is no longer as frightening, because there is more distance.

Attached to emotions

Feeling and emotion are two ideas that are often confused with each other. Every feeling is a message from our true self that brings us in contact with ourselves, while emotions lead us away from that. When we are emotional, we have the tendency to blame others, while with feeling, we take responsibility on ourselves. Feeling overflowing with emotions can be compared to falling into a washing machine and being thrown to all sides without knowing what is happening. But being in touch with your feelings is comparable to standing outside the machine and looking at a spinning wash. You stay with it with-out being in the washing machine. If we are living from our limited self, emotions will keep on flowing over us; however, the person who lives from her true self is in touch with her feelings.

> Hanna: "If I tell my mother something that touches me deeply, she quickly takes off with it. She becomes emotional and I have

the feeling that I have to comfort her, while all I need is for her to listen to me. Basically, I can't experience any connection when she is crying. As a result, now I tend to have only small talk with her."

Hanna feels that she has to take care of her mother when her mother gets emotional. Hanna doesn't feel heard. There are people who can express emotions without changing anything. The reason could be that they became attached to that emotion, to rely on it as a trusted friend. It may also have become a habitual way of trying to interact or to get attention. This can happen on a subconscious level. When I deal with people who are attached to certain emotions, I do not reinforce these emotions by using mind-body therapy. I think that is absolutely pointless. Attachment must step back so that you are no longer blinded by your emotions. If you feel that your emotions are running away with you, pay attention to your body, to your breathing, for instance.

That way, you see what is going on in your body and you can relax. Writing can also be a way to get more distance. Often I see that clients have a tendency to search for explanations for their pain. "Why am I angry, sad, afraid and so on?" This sort of thinking prevents them from feeling the pain and expressing it. I interrupt this process by telling them that for now they don't have to understand what upsets them but they are allowed to feel it.

I stimulated Allie, for example, to increase her frustration by saying as angrily as possible, "I don't know," while stamping her feet at the same time. By doing this, she faced her underlying fear of failure.

In the meantime, Hanna has got up the courage to express her anger to her mother. In that way, Hanna, who during puberty was not given enough space to develop her personality, was able later in life to catch up with this phase. She disengaged herself and created her own life.

Old wounds

> Renate: "Until recently, I often reacted like the wounded child in myself. If someone said something to me, I immediately reacted with indignation, or flattery or burst into tears, without asking myself what was actually intended by the remark. Now I consciously make contact with the adult woman in myself and I ask questions like: 'What do you precisely mean by always, never, again or stupid? What is your need? What are you trying to achieve with that remark?' I feel much more comfortable now that I do this."

Do you recognize the moment that you suddenly change from an adult woman into a vulnerable little girl? This hurt child can suddenly manifest itself in the most unexpected ways. In this way, someone who felt unsafe, didn't have enough freedom or was unappreciated in the past will, as an adult, quickly react like an insecure, angry, sad child as soon as someone starts to criticize, threaten or make a nasty remark. Many people experience events as adults in the same way as they did in their childhood and they react "like a little child."

In other words, they look at the world through the eyes of the child they once were. If we suddenly experience unpleasant feelings when we are in contact with others, are watching a movie, having a dream or reading something, it is possible this has to do with old wounds.

Examples are:

- You promptly feel deserted when an appointment is cancelled.

- Someone is criticizing you and you feel terribly hurt.

- You feel guilty because you made someone angry.

- You are afraid that you are not welcome in a group when your name is not specifically mentioned.

- You are terribly afraid your partner will leave you.

- You feel rejected if he doesn't want to do what you want.

- You feel insecure and sad if your partner acts detached while you are longing for attention.

- You feel trapped and powerless when someone asks you something.

I don't particularly want to dig deep into the past of clients, but looking at the past is meaningful if you want to gain insight into the causes of the feelings that I have described above. I often hear that people are afraid to let themselves feel the pain of old wounds because they have the idea that it will never stop. But if you can find the courage to allow it in, the pain will eventually fade away.

This was the case with Christina. She told me during a session that she wanted to focus on a theme from the past. It had to do with an uncle with whom she had not had contact for years. She told me that he had been her favorite uncle whom she trusted implicitly. He always listened to her, and was logically the first person to whom she confessed, on the phone, that she had bulimia To her horror, it seemed that he had too much to drink at that moment and he confessed that he was in love with her. Now she had a new problem! She felt desperate, she broke off all contact with him and did not tell any one about this dubious situation. But when, twenty years later, she had a nightmare about this, it became clear to her that there was still an old wound. As an adult, she was now capable of looking reality in the eye and handling the pain that she could not admit as a teenager. Now, she fully allowed this pain to come to the surface, stayed with it and registered physical reactions, like tightness of the chest, cold hands and a pounding heart. She knew: this is not now, "it is about pain from the past that is locked in my body." She had to let go of herself completely in order to let go of this pain from the past. As long as you are not conscious of what is going on inside yourself, you live life asleep. The consciousness training is based on learning to observe your thoughts and your feelings. To observe your feelings means that you listen to the little signals of your body. In contact with your true self, you experience the feelings of the here-and-now completely (otherwise you are not living in the here-and-now and chances are that you deny needs and escape into binge eating) and you decide to do something about it or not. From this adult consciousness, you take full responsibility for your thoughts, feelings and behavior. The more conscious you are of your present feelings, the more easily you will be able to give way to pain from the past and to stay with it, without being overwhelmed by it. All feelings, even the "negative ones," are a part of life. If we constantly deny or repress them, we will block ourselves more and more, so that there is no room for positive feelings. If you deny them ("I am not angry") or fight them ("I don't want to feel sad") then you allow these feelings more room than necessary. By, for instance, admitting anger, you will feel it slowly fade from your body.

By allowing ourselves to feel, we can discover what those feelings have to tell us and the negative ones will disappear more quickly than when we repress them. There is nothing we can repress completely. The repressed things will show themselves somewhere else, often disguised. Restlessness,, a feeling of numbness or mortal fear is mostly a reaction to events from the past.

We can experience positive feelings only if we allow ourselves to heal emotional wounds. That doesn't mean that you will never again feel certain wounds. I compare this with a physical wound. Although it healed it will leave a scar. Although you don't feel pain anymore, a scar like that can suddenly hurt on occasion. That will remind you of the painful situation when the wound came into existence. Each human being is damaged to a certain degree, but what will make it worse is if we keep carrying around that damage.

If you never took action to process that pain, it will stay with you. Although you don't think of it consciously, it influences your daily life. It is important that you (if necessary, with professional support) make peace with yourself and start a new chapter.

Let go of illusions

Some time ago, Rianne told me that her ninth therapist wasn't prepared to take a dive into the past with her. The therapist wanted to start from the present and Rianne quickly rejected that. She thought that she had bad luck again. She didn't want to see that there was nothing to gain from the past. Rianne preferred to identify herself as "poor-me." If you want to know joy, you have to accept sorrow. To be an adult means to accept life as it really is. Then we are no longer running away from painful feelings, but we look ourselves in the eye. Many people with compulsive eating behavior have problems in accepting life as it is. The limited I (the hurt child) still wants to believe in fairy tales. She thinks that total happiness will be at her feet when she finally reaches her ideal weight. She hopes that the compulsive eating behavior will go away by itself when she finally meets the ideal partner or finds the perfect job, or owns that dream house.

That is all illusion! The choices you make define your life. If you want to gain control of your own life, you have to look at the world through the eyes of the adult you are right now. What you observe should no longer be biased by experiences from the past. It must show the present as it is. That brings power.

> Diana: "For years I tried very hard to change my father, but nothing worked. On the contrary, it drove us further apart and I felt frustrated by it. My expectations never turned out. Through the training it became clear to me that I had to accept the fact that my father wasn't perfect."

Diana's father is not responsible for his daughter's state of mind, she alone is responsible for that. Painful emotions like Diana's make clear that the problem comes from unfulfilled childhood needs. That doesn't mean that we have to deny these needs or to reject them, but we will only set ourselves right with our past when we accept the harsh reality. Diana realized through the session that her own striving for perfection was an illusion. She started to wonder: When will the cup be full? How much is enough after all these years? Finally she decided to let go of the illusion of perfection and she told herself: I am not disgusting, ugly and bad. I will climb out of the mire.

If I look at the people I coached during this process, I don't see bad, ugly or disgusting people. On the contrary, they have suffered long enough. They are not responsible for what had happened to them, but they are responsible for what they are doing now.

The quality of our life is defined by how we deal with our wounds. We can let our life be defined by these wounds or we can draw power from them.

Exercise: the hot air balloon

Sit in a comfortable position and close your eyes. Concentrate on your breathing without changing it. Imagine that you are in a hot air balloon and keep throwing a sack overboard that holds polluting experiences and poisons: excess baggage that you have carried with you for years. What would you like to throw overboard? How does your body react to this intensive cleaning? The more you throw out, the more you become clean physically and mentally and get a picture of who you really are.

Family entanglements

Without roots no wings.

The family system

> Claudette: "My mother ate when she was angry or sad or lonely. We invariably ate problems away. This was apparently the way to deal with life."

Because of my work, it became clear to me years ago about how many family patterns are passed on generation after generation. Each family member leaves "tracks" behind for the next generation. It looks as if when we have not healed our wounds, we subconsciously pass them on to our offspring. Often-heard statements:

There is always tension in our home.

There is something unspoken in our family that bothers me.

My mother, my sisters and I are extremely afraid.

I have no place in this family, I am an outsider.

A quarter of a century ago the family was often involved in therapy, but at a certain time that became less common. The famous German psychotherapist Bert Hellinger (1925) brought the influence of the family back into the picture. Professionals like psychiatrists, psychologists and physicians started to immerse themselves in this new, deeply influential and quickly growing therapeutic approach. After years of observation, Hellinger discovered that there are certain continual patterns; some examples are: everyone is entitled to a place in the system; in each system there is an order of precedence and there is a balance in giving and taking. This natural order is disturbed when someone is left out. That can have a deep effect within the family system, one that can extend to following generations. By intense loyalty to other family members, at a subconscious level, it seems that the members restore the balance within the family. By means of destined solidarity, it seems that far-reaching events from the past still affect our present life. History can repeat itself if we subconsciously take over the painful fate of a former family member. If this is not cleared up, serious mental and physical problems can result.

I carry the burden for you

We are often willing to give more to our parents than we realize. If your mother is overweight, you can sympathize with her on a subconscious level and become overweight yourself. Or if your mother is dieting, you sympathize by dieting, because otherwise you feel sorry for her. It can work the other way too: what your mother can't do, you do. An example is a client who exercises compulsively. During our first meeting she let me know that she told herself that she had to exercise at least three hours a day. When I asked questions about her family history, it turned out that her mother had a hereditary heart disease and, as a consequence, was not allowed to exercise at all.

Was the reason for this exercising to burn calories only, or was this client also doing it for her mother out of subconscious loyalty?

The natural order is that parents give and children take. Ask, for instance, a child to comfort you, then the roles become reversed.

A girlfriend of mine told me that she comforted her three-year-old son when he fell. Later, she acted as if she wanted to be comforted, too. He said indignantly, "No Mama, I can't do that because you're big and I'm little." Instinctively this little guy understood that that is as unnatural as when water flows upstream. When (sub) consciously a child out of love takes over the role of the parent, it is called parentification. This means that the child wants to take care of the parent, which is unnatural from the position of the child. This leads to fundamental entanglements, and can have a negative influence on relationships in the future.

An example of the consequence of assuming the role of the parent is provided by Lilianne, who always took on responsibilities for everyone, both at her job and in her private life, so that she became completely exhausted. This carrying of others' burdens' started early in her life when Lilianne, as the oldest child, adopted the role of her mother, who had an alcohol problem. Lilianne felt that her mother labored under a heavy burden and, out of love, tried to carry it for her. Bert Hellinger, however, believes that every human is capable of coping with his own destiny. This dignity gives us power. During an individual session it became clear to Lilianne that out of love she had taken over her mother's burdens, but that it was time now to give those burdens back to her. I represented her mother when Lillian gave me a stone that symbolized her heavy burden. With this symbolic act, she also gave her mother her dignity back.

> Lilianne: "Working and the thing with food seemed to be an escape from the pain and emptiness that originated from the past. The session worked to bring an unprecedented liberation. I notice that I now recognize my boundaries and know where to set them. I divide my time in a way to keep my energy on an even level. Also, this has improved my relationship."

When a child is carrying the burden of a parent, it loses, consciously or subconsciously, respect for the parent. Lilianne acted as her mother's mother. This weakens the position of the parent as well as that of the child. This pattern continued in her work and in her relationships. Lilianne noticed that she had a continual tendency to give, but had problems with receiving.

The path from animosity to reconciliation

Angie: "I hate my mother and I am deeply ashamed of her. She only thinks of herself and she boozes. She can't stand being alone, so she makes sure that there is always a man who will take care of her."

After finishing the training Angie started thinking differently about her mother:

"I was a lot like my mother. I didn't booze, but I escaped in binge eating. With that I filled the emptiness, because I also couldn't stand to be alone. I can see now how my mother is suffering, but also that she has to follow her own path. That gives me a free feeling. Now, I feel accepting and generous toward her."

To be an adult doesn't mean to see only yourself as you are, but also to see your parents as they are. Normally, this process passes through a couple of phases. As a child, you think that your parents are completely there for you, then at a certain moment you notice that your parents have shortcomings. You cut yourself off and keep them at a distance.

In the next phase you look for rapprochement. In the last phase reconciliation takes place. You accept your parents as they are. When, however, there are family entanglements, children can (often subconsciously) dissociate themselves from their parents to protect themselves against a heavy burden. This keeps them from treading the natural path from animosity to reconciliation. We all meet in our lives sad, painful and unjust things that are not our fault, but we are responsible for the way we deal with them. Life is not perfect and parents are certainly not perfect. No parent can do everything the right way. If we can look upon our parents and our ancestors as people who are the product of their circumstances, then we can put our life in a broader framework. When we have dealt with painful memories from childhood and examined our childhood patterns, then we will rediscover our true self. Angie, now with an adult and mature insight, was able to see herself and her mother in a new light.

Every relationship, with parents or with someone else, you can look at as an opportunity to get to know yourself better and to become a more liberated human being. Finally, I want to emphasize again that it is true that family entanglements can play a role in an eating problem, but, as I have pointed out in the first chapter, the cause is almost always a combination of different factors. However, this point of view, which according to the founder works in the deepest layers of the subconscious, can offer new perspectives. [8]

Exercise: to receive gifts

Sit in a comfortable position, relax and close your eyes. Imagine that one of your parents is present and that you receive a gift that gives you power. Feel what this means to you. Imagine further that the other parent appears to you and also has a gift. Feel again what this means to you, whatever it was that happened between you, from connection with their true self they wish you well. Say goodbye to them in your own way.

Forgiving

forgiving brings freedom.

No longer holding the other responsible for the way you feel

It is important to forgive and let go of the past in order to heal an eating disorder. In the Greek language, to forgive means literally "to release," saying that you no longer carry with you the burden of an experience. What comes before this is the willingness to let go. A frequent misunderstanding is that the other has to forgive you. Chances are that the other doesn't know anything about this and so makes no gesture towards you. If you go on waiting for this, it will keep taking energy, unless you realize that you are not dependent on the other who will perhaps never express regret.

The person that does not forgive, knows no inner peace of mind. To forgive means setting yourself free. It is an inner cleaning-process. To forgive is a choice. To listen to that choice is a deed of self-love.

An outstanding example is Nelson Mandela, who was in prison for 27 years. I can remember an interview in which he said that he had no feelings of hatred towards his oppressors. All those years he had had time to think. He said that he had banished all the pain and anger, because after being released he wanted consciously to use his energy to bring about changes in South Africa. Unlike the example of Mandela, suffering often exists because of childish, irrational expectations regarding others. Many people have the tendency to hold the other responsible for their unfulfilled longings. Forgiveness challenges you to look inside yourself to find the cause of your irrational expectations, judgments, anger or irritation. You can compare it with dark sunglasses that you put on every day that obscure everything. How realistic is it to expect the other to have the same view of the world as you? To forgive is to make the decision to stop this and to no longer hold the other responsible for how you feel:

> An example by Odette: "After that one remark by my boss I was so disappointed in her that I preferred to leave and never come back again. Promptly, I ate my frustration away. During the session, I found out that my anger had nothing to do with her, but with old wounds regarding my mother.

It takes courage to stop accusing the other and to look at your own actions and ask yourself what you have to learn from it. Odette felt, in the first instance, deeply hurt by the remark from her boss, until she realized that her own interpretation of it was the basis of it. In the chapter "Emotional Detoxification," I wrote that others are capable of bringing our old pain to the surface. This means we are often irritated by people who actually have nothing to do with this irritation. That was the case here.

Odette forgave herself for again letting her imagination run wild, but what relieved her the most was that, thanks to this incident with her boss, she could let go of old pain. To forgive is not an outward action, it is a process in which you look inside. You suffer from your pain, your anger and your judgments, not because of the one who hurt you, but because of what you did to yourself. So there lies the necessity for forgiveness. Because Odette forgave herself, she not only freed herself, but she also freed her boss from the image she had made of her.

Carla: "I suffered for years because of my ex-partner's addiction to alcohol. For a long time I pretended it was not that bad. Then came the shame and intense hatred towards him. After the divorce, I gradually came to look the harsh reality in the eye. Now I am at the point that I accept him as he is."

How painful this can be, forgiving starts with accepting the facts. If you look reality in the eye and no longer fight against it, then forgiveness has a chance. Not the one who is hated, but the one who hates, is putting itself in prison and has the most problems with it. To not forgive is to poison yourself. The antidote is forgiveness. As long as you put the blame on the other, you will be the victim. To be able to forgive, it is important to step out of the role of victim. With this you stop accusing the other and you stand on your own strength. You can leave the trouble you have been through behind, unless you think you haven't yet suffered enough.

If someone did you wrong, you can bear a very heavy burden, but you are not your past. What limitation did you put on yourself as a result of this event? How does it feel when you imagine that you are free of pain, anger, rancor and guilt?

You can let yourself be consumed by the past or you can decide to start a new chapter.

How can you forgive yourself?

Not only can we feel that we got the short end of the stick, but we can also be frustrated because we are not living up to an idealized image. We can feel guilty about all kinds of things. It can happen after eating a banana as an in-between snack, although the "healthy thinker" knows this is nonsense. Maybe you have the tendency to feel guilty about things you did in the past, but you can't change that now. The critic in you says: you could have done it better. But, like everyone else, you are not perfect. When we forgive ourselves unconditionally, we can award ourselves the right to be a human who has normal shortcomings and weaknesses. Are you going to put things that have happened in the past behind you? A new life starts when you forgive yourself. This step toward self-love is one of the most important steps you can take to heal yourself. Years ago I once read something about forgiveness, and suddenly I realized that if there was one person in my life I had to forgive, it was myself. I allowed the pain in and I forgave myself for all those years that I wasn't capable of accepting myself as I am. I forgave myself for failing both myself and those around me. I mourned for the irretrievable past. After that I had an enormous feeling of liberation and deep calm.

Through true forgiveness you can put an end to years of suffering once and for all. My experience is that for many people forgiveness is difficult, and so the chances are great that binge eating will continue to exist. To not cherish rancor is a choice. We can always draw upon the source of forgiveness if we are flexible and willing.

Exercise: forgiving yourself

The first step toward forgiving is to be willing to forgive yourself. After that, is to dare to allow the pain in and let go of expectations. After all, you have to open your heart, so that love can flow.

1. What were you incapable of forgiving yourself for? Start with a little incident. If more things pop up, choose only one. Keep track of the things in your life that you could change if you can forgive yourself for this. How do you look at yourself then? What are you saying to yourself then? How does that feel? There is always a choice between being a victim and being in charge of your own life. If you choose the latter, take action. Make an appointment with yourself in the near future when you are going to take the next step, or take it now.

2. Make contact as an adult woman with the "wounded child" in you and completely allow in the painful feelings arising from this situation. Feelings will bring you to your true self, while emotions lead you away from it. Do this without losing yourself in it (as is described earlier at "Emotional Detoxification").

3. The last step in this process of freeing yourself is to imagine that you fill your heart with love. Imagine further that this healing energy flows from your heart to every part of your body that needs it. If you now look at the respective situation from your true self, you can feel acceptance and compassion. Feel the freedom that radiates from this.

Probably, the experience is different now than it was in the beginning. If that is not the case, then it is possible that your "limited self" is in the way. (Maybe the powerless-one, the bossy-one or the critical-one.) In that case you know what to do (see chapter 2). The more you do this exercise, the more you will start to feel free and energetic.

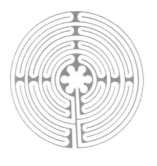

COMING HOME

7

LIVING A FULL LIFE

Living from your heart is living in full.

Coming home to yourself.

Coming home to yourself is to be at peace with yourself.

Introduction

In chapter 1 (see "The process of overeating to living in full") I wrote about the labyrinth as a symbol of the path to self-liberation and the phases we go through to achieve this. During the second phase you make the transition from childhood (limited self) to an adult existence (your true self). You look at the past with different eyes now. There is compassion for yourself and your environment. You reconciled with your circumstances in life. There is purification and gratitude. The path through the labyrinth has led you to your centre. The treasure you find there is who you essentially are. You are not the person you became, you are who you really are deep down inside. You feel reborn.

> Mary Kay's dream: "I am climbing a very narrow spiral staircase, like one you could find in a castle. The staircase is so narrow that I can hardly pass my body through it. It seems that this stair is tailor made. The passage is dark and narrow, but I keep on climbing. Then I finally see the last step. From one moment to the next I'm suddenly standing in the light and I have a splendid view. I am naked and feel free."

Self-esteem and self-confidence

Years ago, I received a farewell gift from one of my clients. It was a cassette with the song "Greatest love of all" by Whitney Houston. This song conveys how you feel when you have come home to yourself. Whitney sings "learning to love yourself, it is the greatest love of all."

Constantly I hear and read how important it is to increase your self-confidence and to gain more self-respect, but all this starts with "the self." In the beginning, most clients hardly know who they are. Someone put this into words: "If I were to be cut open, nothing would be left of me, because there is nothing on the inside." This woman looked upon herself as nothing more than an empty shell. As a result of a loving construction of the self a sense of self-esteem and self-confidence will develop, naturally. The inner journey can be summed up as a search for your true self. If we live from this perspective we will find out what our preferences and passions are. Out of your true self you give your own answer and you let your own song be heard. A dream and a quotation, both by Irene:

"I dream that a choir is standing on the platform in a large church. Fascinated, I listen to the music which sounds heavenly. After the break, it seems I am supposed sing a solo. I am scared to death, but I do it.

Step by step I showed my true face, no longer pretended that everything was fine, but allowed myself to be vulnerable. I no longer abandoned myself, but brought my feelings and needs out into the open. As a result, I no longer needed compensatory behavior in the form of binge eating. Some people disappeared out of my life, but they were the ones that I called 'energy-gluttons.' So, looking back, I wasn't sorry about losing them. The friends who are a part of my life now are the ones with whom I can completely be myself and vice versa. I hear that they feel that way about me, too. These beloved friendships are based on equality and mutual respect. I can embrace myself now and truly say that I love myself."

Binge eating or other escape behavior keeps us in prison, if we hold on to a false self-image. Feeling inferior is completely the opposite of self-love. There is no reason to feel inferior, nobody in the world is like you: you are unique! You are fine because of who you are, not because of what you do. Self-awareness is the basis of being in the world. In contact with our true self we no longer play hide and seek with ourselves and our surrounding: we stay faithful to ourselves.

From saboteur to companion

Anna's dream: "I am on my way to get some groceries. Suddenly, my path is obstructed by three wolves. I am terribly frightened, but instinctively I know what to do. I start to softly caress them and my fear disappears completely. The wolves enjoy this unexpected attention and are like putty in my hands."

Everything we deny becomes our shadow. What we fight against, continues to exist. Darkness doesn't disappear by fighting it, but by lovingly shining a light on it. That means making oneself familiar with the opposing forces in ourselves and making peace with them. Healing depends on recognition, acknowledgement and integration of our shadow side, or the non-radiant part of our self.

Living in full means taking responsibility for our radiance and our lack of radiance! Through consciousness training clients see the world more and more as it really is. They don't take the things to heart that heavily anymore. So, the other that seems to want to harm them is no longer a monster. They can also look at their inner monster without judgment. Because of this, the unripe, fearful and sabotaging element that kept them in prison can heal. They realize: I am not who I thought I was, and they finally find themselves again. The gorge-monster was on a search for happiness outside itself; it did not know that it can only be found within ourselves. Maybe it was originally "the comforter," (and at a certain moment went totally berserk through all that eating), or it stands for the need for relaxation. When we find out what this saboteur stands for, we can properly satisfy the following needs: comfort, relaxation, letting our hair down and the need to be rewarded. Instead of ruling it can serve.

> Andrea wrote: "After doing the exercise I was quietly enjoying the afterglow and I felt satisfied. And then there was that inner voice again that destroys so much, that always wants me to be, think, feel different, always criticizes me, makes me look ridiculous, my devil. My good feeling vanished. The "what-would-they-think-of-me" shame was there again. Suddenly something happened. I looked at my devil, I imagined that I reached out my arms and embraced him and whispered: "And I love you too." Without my knowing where it came from, suddenly all this love was flowing through me. I felt myself opening up and the flow of love increase in intensity. The devil became a little devil, smaller and smaller, and let out its last little peeps. But when I kept embracing him, during which my warm feeling for him continued, he disappeared . . . and with that all the negative . . . I was perfectly happy and being so deeply moved, I cried silently. I embraced myself completely and I experienced unconditional happiness."

Exercise: embracing your shadow

Go to your little retreat. Close your eyes and concentrate on your breathing. Next recall a moment in which you felt love. Take this feeling in completely. Look from within your true self with compassion at the saboteur. Place that wounded part of you in the light and wrap it in love. Then imagine that the negative feeling dissolves by itself in your love.

Life as a learning school

Happiness is not to be found in the things
themselves but in how I experience them.

Introduction

The last part of this book deals with the third and final phase, in which clients have left the labyrinth. The caterpillar has become a butterfly. The old is transformed into the new. You realize that you are endlessly more than your body, your thoughts and feelings. If you have walked this path you feel that your attitude to life has changed. What you need is not what you thought you needed. You thought you would find happiness in eating, even though you felt lost deep down inside. Now you realize that you can find the source of satisfaction, fulfillment and joy within yourself. What used to be your problem, has now led you to a new existence.

> Eva: "I was a professional dancer, but because of bulimia I became very ill and could no longer dance. I decided to stop for awhile. When I was doing all right again I discovered that my old job wasn't right for me anymore. I wanted to start a family more than anything. I now have a partner and gave birth to two children and I work at home. Dancing had become something

I do for fun, for instance when I go to a disco. Also I take salsa
lessons. In this way I found my niche in life."

Eva asked herself: What do I really want? Because she connected
with the core of her being, she was capable of making choices that
were in harmony with her deepest wishes. Moreover, she stayed
faithful to herself.

From fear of life to solidarity with the earth

Maya: "When I realized that eating is a confirmation of life
on the deepest level, I suddenly realized that the problems I
used to have with food (starting from the day I was born) were
probably a protest against living on earth on a subconscious
level. I neither felt at home on earth nor in my body. I was only
happy when I was surrounded by nature, there I felt connected
to the universe. As a little girl I called this separation in myself
'homesick for heaven.' I didn't want to feel the pain that life on
earth inevitably brings with it and I started to avoid that in all
possible ways. Only when after years of neglecting my body I
suddenly looked death in the eye, did I consciously choose to
be here."

Eating is the most fundamental expression of life. By eating we
connect ourselves with this earthly existence. With this we make a
choice to live, time and again. If we consciously connect ourselves
with the earth we say yes completely to life and we are prepared
to accept the fact that life along with joy and love also brings pain
and sorrow.

Millicent: "Even as a child I had the feeling that I would break
down under all the responsibilities that are just a part of life.
I've left the illusion behind that I had to save the whole world,
along with the irrational idea that someone could bear my

burden. I am standing on my own two feet now and they are capable of carrying me. I can do it!"

Many people have a longing, deep inside them, for an ideal father or mother (or prince charming) which will make all their problems vanish into thin air. Of course, this longing stays unfulfilled. The reality is that we have to take care of ourselves. If we simply acknowledge and discover that all we need is present in ourselves, we can stand in the world with inner strength and self-confidence.

To feed yourself is to become internally powerful. After a period of time, clients come to realize more and more they can be their own archetype mother. They feel that they are capable of enveloping themselves in loving devotion. They trust their own possibilities and live life on their own conditions. They no longer deny their inner knowledge, but turn it into actions because they believe in their own power.

The silver lining around the dark cloud

> Maria: "I asked Joanna why I had to deal with all this suffering. She suggested I ask 'the wise-one' with whom I had made contact before. This voice said: 'To learn from.' Suddenly a deep calm came over me."

Regularly, I am asked questions like: What is the meaning of all this? According to the great spiritual leaders, there is but one important question: What is the purpose of life on earth?

We are here to get to know ourselves and to develop ourselves. I look at life as one big school. Sometimes, I literally dream that I am back in school again. I know now that in this way it is being made clear to me that I have to learn one thing and another in this "school of life." If we remind ourselves that we are on earth to learn life-lessons, then we are capable in difficult situations of asking ourselves the question: "What could I learn from this experience?" instead of

"Why does this always have to happen to me?" Most people think life is hard and that is not surprising, because, superficially speaking, life can appear to be a senseless chaos. But, on a deeper level, you can see the whole and experience the meaning of life. That can give you just that extra support to understand the meaning of your existence. When I had to write my resume for a training course I didn't look at myself as a powerless victim who saw her life as a series of uncorrelated events, but I saw painful events as a learning experience that life offered me. Tragedies appeared to be blessings in disguise. However, I didn't have that insight when I was still struggling with my eating disorder. The reason why someone develops an eating problem is hard to find out, but, often afterwards, clients state that it is an enrichment. To find out what kind of positive aspects an eating disorder has produced, there first has to be acknowledgement of the negative aspects. When we give it a place in our lives, it will bring new aspects of ourselves to the surface.

> Kitty: "My husband died suddenly. Life had no meaning for me anymore. I felt numb for a long time. Now I am capable of looking reality in the face. He is dead and I am alive. I have to go on, no matter how painful it is. Through this process of mourning I started to look at life differently. The quality of life is worth more than earning money. I finally gave myself time for hobbies after all those years. Through the death of my husband I found out who my true friends were. Keeping in touch with these people is worth more than anything else in the world."

Psychiatrist Victor Frankl discovered his power and that of his fellow prisoners when he was in a concentration camp during World War II. He recognized that it is not so much what we expect from life, but what life expects from us. This conviction became the core of his life's work. Not only Frankl and his fellow prisoners, but everyone who has achieved the journey through the labyrinth and with that freed himself, is a true hero.

Clients try in their own way to discover a tapestry in their lives, by which not only their eating problem, but also other far-reaching events become meaningful. These people are capable of rising above their misery. The power of life lies in the ability to heal the wounds that we sustain.

Suffering can create and develop new characteristics. This situation not only requires courage, but also trust, flexibility, directness and the ability to put things into perspective. Clients like Kitty are able to discover the silver lining behind the dark cloud. They have become stronger, have more self-confidence and are thankful for the good things in their lives, which, as a result, have more depth. The path that we follow on earth is paved with life-lessons. Until our death, we have to go through ordeals. Our development depends on the willingness to learn lessons and to integrate them into our daily lives. By learning these daily lessons we come more and more in contact with our true self. A growing consciousness leads to more confidence in our internal knowledge, which helps many people to feel that more and more they are becoming a part of the universal source of power that binds us together.

Self-actualization

Most of the time your obsession with food is only a symbol of your true longings. We hunger for a fulfilled existence. The meaning of life is the deeper feeding of heart and soul. If we get the best out of ourselves, we give meaning to our existence. Then we no longer live to eat, but we eat to live. The Indian philosopher, Patanjali, says that when you let yourself be inspired by an ambitious goal, a special project, all your thoughts become free; your spirit becomes free from all limitations, your consciousness expands and you enter a big, new, wonderful world. Dormant powers, gifts and talents awaken and you discover that there is more in you than you had ever imagined.[9]

The possibilities of one human will never be found in another, because every person is unique. At birth everyone brings certain gifts on which his life can later be built, but we ourselves can choose whether to use them or not. It may seem attractive to win the lottery, or to be sent home with a golden handshake and have a permanent vacation, but this kind of fantasy is an escape from daily life.

Research shows that most people are not happy when they are doing something that they believe to be meaningless and they are equally unhappy when they don't have to do anything at all. But people feel happy when they can lose themselves in realizing a self-chosen goal (big or small). That gives meaning to their existence. Naturally, no one is saying that you should become a hopeless perfectionist, trying desperately to get the best out of yourself. On the contrary, it is important that you find out what you enjoy and what makes you happy— in other words, do what is in keeping with your talents. There are challenges that can be realized, like having a child, taking a certain course of studies, or doing volunteer work. If service comes from your heart, it doesn't feel like a duty or an obligation. When you look around you, you will see those inspired people immediately. They do "their thing." They bring out their soul and radiate a strong zest for life. We don't live our dreams by waiting until we reach our goal, but by enjoying every moment of the process. Clarissa, who had left her job and was in a phase of reorientation, wrote:

> "What I need the most at this moment is silence, which gives me so much peace. In my thoughts I'm going on a voyage of discovery and a question arises: Who am I? What are my needs? What gives my life meaning? Basically, I am teaching myself to coach and that is an interesting process. It is not vague or weird."

Although at a certain moment it is clear what suits you, insecurity may suddenly sneak up on you. Janet told me, a little tensely, that she had responded to a vacancy that seemed made for her. The

next day she was going to have a job interview. She fit the require-
ments perfectly and hoped with all her heart that she would be
hired, but suddenly she heard that old little voice again: "You are
not good enough."

I invited her to contact "the wise-one."

> "During the visualization I asked the wise-one: 'Is it okay to be
> the way I am?'
>
> 'Of course,' he said. Right away I started to laugh at myself.
> 'What am I getting so stressed out about? If they don't want me,
> it doesn't change who I am. I am okay,' and with that attitude I
> am going to have the interview."
>
> (And Janet got the job.)

Your true self will never expect something from you that you
can't do. If you quietly ask yourself the question what you love
most, and what you care about in life, then the answer will come by
itself. That can't happen any other way, because in your innermost
being lies the true answer.

You are being touched from the inside, and not by something
temporary. From this deep knowledge you draw the power to handle what is needed. Other sources of help with this are: listening to
your dreams, listening to your suggestions, reading a book, watching a movie that suddenly gives you insight, listening to a song or
a poem, or talking to a person who says something enlightening.
In the next sub-chapter (Surrender) I will go into this more deeply.
We have unlimited possibilities. It seems we only use about 20%
of these. Life challenges us to make use of that potential. We can
do much more than we think we can. Limitations are in our mind,
the well-known sabotaging thoughts. Isn't it true that your life is
meaningful and that you were born to use your talents?

Exercise: the rose

Close your eyes. Concentrate on your breathing without changing it. Imagine yourself as a rose in the bud. The leaves unfold themselves one by one until the flower is completely opened. Then the heart becomes visible in which there is a kernel of pure light. When you inhale, you let the light come in and when you exhale, it radiates to all sides.

Surrender

The man who lives his live in surrender,
will experience help at crucial moments.

Introduction

Full of enthusiasm, I wanted to start writing this section, when I came down with a bad case of the flu. I was in bed with a fever, but could see quickly the humor of it. This was a lesson in surrendering. I had to deliver my manuscript before a certain date and suddenly there appeared this little angel disguised as a little devil. You can't push the river. I had been very busy and deep inside I just wanted to catch my breath. So, very confident, I relaxed, enjoyed the unexpected rest and it turned out that I still had enough time. Surrendering doesn't mean that you escape from daily life, but just dive into it more deeply.

You stay anchored in yourself while you follow your deepest impulses without asking where it will lead you. You offer yourself with all that is in you. Then you live life to the fullest and your existence is one big adventure.

Then it turns out that you can do much more than you ever thought. Surrender and fear can't exist at the same time. It is a skill to stay in touch with your stream of life. Surrender is to trust that it will turn out right for you, although that trust is sometimes hidden under a thick layer of dust. You will uncover it when you are in touch with your inborn wisdom. One who lives in surrender, will find help at crucial moments.

Many people run away from inner emptiness, but the pain dissolves if we dare to surrender completely to the emptiness. I had that experience when I learned that my father had suddenly passed away. I was alone at that moment, my partner was in a foreign country. Family and close friends offered to be with me, but however tempting this offer seemed, I knew that I had to be alone. The emptiness that I felt at that moment I did not want to eat away as I had done in the past, nor did I want to fill it with the presence of loved ones. I had to go through it alone. When I opened up to this completely, it turned out that I didn't feel lonely or lost: slowly but surely the emptiness filled itself. I felt peaceful. Stronger than ever I felt oneness and deep solidarity with my true nature. It turned out I was my best company!

Trusting internal guidance

Our true self points out the way in the search for wholeness. Internal leadership takes us to our destiny, back to our essence. If we listen to this source of wisdom we know what to do and what not to do. We are part of an endless field of force that is always at our disposal. It sends us messages in the form of dreams, bodily sensations like goose bumps, but also spontaneous suggestions, a sudden memory, a phone call, a movie that unexpectedly gives insight or a book that you open at the right page.

Terri told me that the words of a little song helped her to go on:

Terri: "After that session, I stepped into the car and I thought: I can't do this anymore. I think it is too much confrontation. I started the car, the radio was playing and immediately I heard the song "No more escaping" by Jenny Arean and Frans Halsema. I cried and laughed at the same time."

Carl Jung, the well-known psychologist, called meaningful accidents "synchronization." To receive such messages we must be tuned in to the correct wavelength. This requires that we be open to a message that can sound different from what we expect. It is very important that you be relaxed with this and that you also wait in trust. If something is not successful and you let it go, then often, afterwards, the solution appears unexpectedly. Trust grows when we dare to leap into the deep and believe profoundly that our true self is leading us. Often, however, we meet our internal dragons (the limited self). Your parents, your partner or your friends can also suddenly change into a dragon, who, with the best intentions in the world, try to protect you from taking what they consider to be a wrong turn.

But the voice of our true self keeps calling . . .

If our true self is not fed, it will withdraw more and more until it becomes no more than a little pilot-light. Just as a plant needs the right conditions to enable it to grow, we get more power of life if we create the right environment to express our original self. This can involve being open to nature, by going to a place that you experience as healing. Other possibilities are candlelight, classical music, literature, poetry, a bath filled with herbs or ethereal oils, and singing, dancing, writing or painting.

There is something bigger than you. We are part of a bigger whole. It is essentially nameless, but part of experience. That means that we don't have to act alone.

When we ask for "higher" intervention, we can take a step back and allow ourselves to symbolically accept the hand of a wise guide or another source of help. (See chapter 3: Soul Food.) When we open ourselves completely to this help, we get answers that we could not think of and solutions offer themselves. You can ask something that is bigger and stronger than you to carry the burden that is too heavy for you. This invisible power is always present. You can think, for instance, of the enormous source of power of the moon and the stars, or perhaps, like my aunt, you prefer to think, "I let it go and let God do his way." Ask aloud for help; then you will be heard.

Dreams as a source of inner guidance

The power of dreams is that they go beyond our limited self. They appear at night when our will is strongly reduced.[10] Then what truly lives inside you becomes visible. For that reason, dreams are important direction indicators. They are a personal document, a letter to yourself with a message. They show you what you are engaged in, what your way of living is and who you are. They point out talents and possibilities. Dreams can be funny, inspiring, but also very confrontational. The things you run up against in every day life, you meet in your dreams. For instance, you are being pursued or you can't find your way home. It is important to pay attention to recurrent dreams and nightmares; the subconscious signals that something is going on.

> Simone: "I had a recurrent nightmare about a tiger who tried to attack me. In my dream the tiger became more and more aggressive. In the beginning, I ran away. After I started the training, to my astonishment, I saw myself at a certain moment turning to hunt the tiger. In the final dream about the tiger, he only wanted to play with me."

We are often asleep to the things that are real in our life. Dreams can wake you up and be a path to insight and healing. Simone had a recurrent nightmare, but as she started to feel more free, this dream theme changed. Every human has dreams, but it is possible that you can't remember them. You can start by putting pen and paper next to your bed. If you have a specific question, you can write it down before you go to sleep. You might say to yourself, a couple of times, that the next morning you will write down everything you can remember, even if it is only a flash. Experience teaches that a single picture can mean a lot. In the long run you will remember more and more. The most important question you can ask yourself is: what touches me the most in the dream and what does the dream invite me to do?

To me, dreams are an important source of internal guidance; if you discover what your resources are, you can call on them in difficult times. Furthermore, you can draw strength from collecting things that bring you into contact with the essence of who you are. This could be a poem, objects from nature, a saying, something you wrote yourself or another wrote to you. Put these together and keep in touch with them. Cherish these treasures in your heart. When you surround yourself with them, they will strengthen and empower you.

Although we are feeling lost, there is always a part of us that still is connected with wholeness. I discovered that dreams can give you a glimpse of something more, when I was suffering from bulimia and dreamed that a treasure was buried in my own garden. It turned out to be the life-elixir, the essence of everything, the circle of life. From my dream report:

In my garden, just beneath the earth, there is a treasure. It is a transparent bottle filled with a clear, neutral-tasting life-water. If I have a problem and I drink only one sip of this elixir (that is only attuned to me), then I am clear-headed and know what to do. After I take such a sip, the bottle fills itself again.

Everyone owns a treasure. When we open ourselves to this inner source, then our path in life will unfold before us.

Exercise: internal guidance

Every time you have an important question, you can write it down and feel confident that you will get an answer. After that, for instance, you can image yourself putting this question in a large box and to close that box by tying it up with a ribbon in your favorite color. Hand this parcel to a higher source of power. You can get an answer in different ways. It can appear spontaneously, while you are writing the question, or it can appear later in the form of an insight. Maybe the answer appears because you react spontaneously to a deep impulse, or it can be that you suddenly imagine that "the wise-one" is talking to you. You can never force an answer, so wait in confidence.

From surviving to living a full life

One who accepts the emptiness, becomes fulfilled.

Who can better put into words how living a fulfilled life feels than those who broke the spell of binge eating? There are quotations from clients that describe the many changes that have to do with self-esteem and self-confidence. These people know from their own experience that life is worthwhile and that it is possible to heal completely from compulsive eating behavior. I hope that their words will help you even more.

Living from your own strength.

> Marissa: "If I compare what I was when I started and what I am now, there are two words that are important: dependence (then) strength (now). When I started, I was like a caged little bird that felt fatigued and miserable, that wanted to be free, but doubted that she could ever find the strength to spread her wings and fly. Gradually, I learned that I am much more powerful than I ever felt before. Somewhere very deep inside I knew it, but I could not feel it anymore. Then I was dependent, sad, fatigued through and through, lonely, imprisoned by my addictions (alcohol and food). Now, most of the time, I am powerful, free to make choices and molding my life, open and happy, energetic, and I live a healthy lifestyle."

Accepting food.

Iris: "First of all, food was the most important thing in my life. Because of this, the time came when I became entangled in an argument with myself. I realized that if I kept going on like this I was going to die. I had to search for my happiness in other things. Now that the magic of it is gone, I realize that the meaning of food is what I think it is."

Responsibility for your own existence:

Claudia: "I gave up the illusion that my parents have to be there for me in the way that I wish them to be. Those old unfulfilled childish needs I left behind. I have reconciled with my parents. They are still the same people, but now I look at them with different eyes. Also, I left behind the illusion that my partner has to make me happy. Those were 'child-wishes.'

I am now at the point that I am responsible for my own existence. I now have the deep knowledge that I can always count on myself, no matter what is happening. I am the captain of my ship."

Be open to intimacy

Alexis: "In the past I did not know real intimacy. I went from one partner to the next. I doubt if I really loved any of them. I don't think so, because I was only occupied with myself. Now, for the first time, I am living with a partner. This partner is the love of my life. He is the first person to whom I really listen. I feel a deep bonding with him, but I think that is because now I dare to completely give myself. For that I had to learn first to accept and love myself. I stuffed away my insecurity about myself for years, now I feel peace."

Looking at people more realistically

Ann: "In the past I had the tendency to divide people into little angels and little devils. The little angels I placed on pedestals. Of course, they all tumbled down one by one, because they were not little angels, but people of flesh and blood, each with his own shortcomings. I always felt disappointed in friendships, until I noticed I created that myself by my unrealistic attitude toward others. I can make jokes about it now, like saying: I was wearing my rose colored glasses again."

Establishing structure

Ruth: "I suffer from manic-depression and I did the training in connection with an eating addiction. I found out that when I eat healthy, I feel much better psychologically. I used to be in utter chaos. Now, among other things, I have learned to bring structure to my life. For instance, I make up a week's menu and go grocery shopping twice a week. I limit the use of sugar and buy food at the organic food store. It is no trouble for me to eat healthy, because now I feel energetic and balanced. Chi-neng qi gong also helps me with that. Because of this, I now have both feet on the ground."

Accepting your own body.

Julia: "For the first time I dared to visit a sauna. In advance I felt very tense about it, but, when I was there, to my astonishment the tension suddenly disappeared. It started to snow. Without thinking about it I ran naked to the enclosed garden and made a round dance on the grass while I felt the sensation of the wet snowflakes on my warm skin. I cried with happiness. Finally I felt free in my body."

Trusting your own feelings and needs.

Rosalie: "I feel vital again! My laundry list of complaints has disappeared. That is not only the result of having a normal and healthy eating pattern again. I feel now what I want. Before that I lived as a surrogate, occupied only with pleasing the other. Now that I know what my needs and my own qualities are, I am also less upset by the rougher sides of life."

Being less dependent on others.

Nadine: "I thought in the past that if only I could have a relationship and live with a partner, I would have no problems anymore. Then I wouldn't have to gorge again, then I'd be happy. So I made myself dependent on my partner, because he had to make me happy. Now I know that nobody can make me happy, Yes, for a while, maybe. But I have to find happiness in myself. I am getting better at it; my relationship has become lighter."

Letting negative thoughts go

Erna: "I can look at it now whenever a negative thought appears again. I realize that it keeps me away from reality, that a thought like that is not my true self. I know now that I have a choice of accepting it or letting go of it. Sometimes I imagine that I am attaching this negative thought to a balloon and sending it up into the air."

Positive body-experience

Frederique: "During the exercise I was asked to draw a picture of my ideal figure. To my astonishment I discovered that suddenly I did not want to be skinny. It turned out I already had my ideal figure. Finally I accepted it and I could say to myself: My body is fine the way it is!"

Finally, the last four letters.

Nina: "When unexpected events in my life piled themselves up in my overflowing backpack, I went through what I had learned in the training to drastically attack this situation. This wasn't easy, the entire confrontation was like holding up a mirror before myself. I found it very healing. For me especially, because I was a difficult person. Afraid of everything, surly and trapped in my shell. The therapy got me out of it and I discovered more things about myself that I liked. So I am not so insecure anymore. Then almost everything in my life was dark, where now the sun is shining brightly. Unexpected events caught me completely off guard, like a feather that can't go any further and that slowly has to turn back so that everything falls into in place. I can say now that I am extremely happy. I can process negative thoughts by expressing them, either verbally, or by crying and so on. Also, I am able now, after processing, to bend them to something positive instead of keeping them inside and muffling them by binge eating. For more than twenty years I have thought that food was my safest friend, while actually it was holding back my development. Now that I no longer have to cope with it compulsively, I realize how I have been set free and how much time I have left over now for the real important things in my life. Because of that, I was ready to start a relationship, something I wasn't ready for in the past. I already had a 'friend,' but that is all far behind me. I can now really speak of a former life and a life in the present."

Nikita: "When I started the training, I was an insecure and frightened little girl. I hated my body and was unhappy. All day I was busy thinking about eating or not eating, and that controlled my life. I am a clever girl, but, because of my concentration problems, I could not get as much out of my studies as I wanted to. I always had many creative hobbies, but they weren't satisfying anymore because I didn't feel good about myself. I suppressed my feelings, and because of that my creativity broke down. Because I was so insecure, I also had problems meeting people. I thought that others were not interested in my company. After a year my life has completely changed. I feel I opened up like a flower. My thoughts about food are mostly limited to 'What are we eating today?' I can concentrate better and I am interested again in a couple of my hobbies. I am more secure about myself and am open to others; I enlarged my circle of friends. On all fronts I am doing much better and others can see that, too. I have a lust for life again and I radiate that. More and more I get compliments and they do me good. I feel now like a woman of the world!"

Mari: "Of course I knew that I didn't handle eating well, but I thought eating was my problem and I didn't think about the underlying problems. When I look back, I see that insecurity and a negative self-image played a big role in my eating disorder. More and more I suffered from binge eating attacks which, in turn, made me feel more and more insecure. I entered a downward spiral in which I doubted myself, my abilities, wondered if people thought I was nice—in short, if I was worth anything. I was always trying to please others and lost myself completely."

A couple of points which I want to list:

- I listen much more to my own needs and know better what I want:

- I am less carried away by ideas and thoughts of others.

- I need less appreciation from others to be proud of myself because I appreciate myself more. I am less self-critical and see my positive qualities.

- I ask less of myself, am more relaxed and peaceful. I can let go more easily.

- I am no longer disappointed in my expectations, because I talk about my needs.

- I was afraid of the emptiness that would ensue if I no longer had an eating problem, but I know now that the opposite is true.

- All kinds of good and valuable things (peace, relaxation, ideas) have returned.

- Because I am now conscious of the inner saboteur, I feel more free, my self-confidence has grown and I dare to do more.

- I am not that easily impressed anymore.

- I have learned not to run away from feelings, but to experience them.

- I have learned to put myself in first place because I am worth it."

Judi: Thanks to the training I have become a happy and complete human being. I know who I am now, I truly love myself and think that I am beautiful. Secretly, I am a little bit glad I had an eating problem. If that had not have been the case, I would never have known what I am like deep down inside and who I really am. I wanted to find peace and quiet in myself and learn how to eat in a normal way. The good part of this period I think is that I learned and discovered much more than I thought was possible, and it was always in a pleasant way. I am more at peace, more lively, more beautiful, and I really mean that! I enjoy what I eat, also that delicious ice-cream, and I don't have to vomit anymore. I think life is wonderful and I don't want to be perfect anymore. I can laugh again, cry and count to ten when I become angry. I love my partner even more, with whom I now enjoy making love. I'm not afraid to have a child anymore. Can take a break when there is a mess and a lot going on, dare to say sorry, don't have to do everything alone anymore. My weight is no longer 80 pounds, I can read a book again, enjoy qi gong and no longer compare myself with others and now love myself. What I liked especially was that different methods were used. I know now what my pitfalls are. I now dare to walk on my own two feet. I can now behave like an adult woman: a woman who likes being an adult and who can leave the child behind. And, sometimes, when I feel like it, I call little Judi to dance around for a short while, and to jump in a puddle, to say hello to life. The adult Judi and the child shake hands and set out together."

By means of periodic follow-ups I see old clients a couple of times a year. Judi recently gave birth to a healthy baby. With this, her deepest wish has been fulfilled.

Be Quiet

You think perhaps
that you have to say something
you think perhaps
that you have to cheer me up
you want perhaps
to see me smile again
and enjoy
you think perhaps that you have to
comfort me
and advise me.
What I ask is this:
do you want to
listen to my story
again and again
to what I feel and think.
You only need to be silent,
to look at me
to give me time.
You don't even need
to understand my sorrow
but if it is possible
just to accept
how it feels for me.
Your listening presence
will make my day different.

(Source: Marinus van den Berg,
Words In Silence, Kok 2000)

221

Exercises

Sometimes, I hear people say that they take in this book just like a binge eating attack: quickly consume it, without really tasting it. Also, I hear sometimes: I read piles of books, why am I not successful in real life? Breaking the spell of binge eating will hardly ever be successful by reading about it. This book challenges you to make time for you to think about yourself, to do the exercises like writing down your thoughts and to work actively on your goals. Read this book anew (also the directions for use) to be sure that you understand the basics. If you make a routine of the exercises, the results will astonish you.

Appendix 1

Suggestions for getting started right away.

New clients often ask if I have tips they can start right away with. Although an eating problem is mostly a symptom of an underlying problem, it is worthwhile to examine it more closely, and the following suggestions can be of help. They are also useful when it looks as if someone is on the verge of have a relapse.

1. An irregular eating pattern provokes binge eating attacks. You increase regularity by eating three times a day at fixed times. Your body will adjust itself to this (biological clock). Do this one step at a time: for instance, start with breakfast; if this goes well, then move on to the next meal. Planning meals offers an overall picture. When you eat regularly and only have one snack in between meals, then there is time to look at what you eat.

2. Avoid, for the time being, alcohol and sugar-rich products. This way you have less chance to start binge eating. Avoid also artificial sweeteners that are to be found in soft drinks. They slow down the digestive system and sustain the need for sweets. Also gradually replace white flour products (white bread, white rice, pasta and the like) with whole grain products.

3. Avoid products containing caffeine, like coffee, black tea, cacao and cola. Caffeine gives a quick energy boost, but lasts only for a short time. It causes a stress-reaction and raises the blood sugar level. Gradually replace coffee with green tea or herb tea.

4. If you are highly sensitive to surrounding stimuli, like the bakery or fast food restaurants, avoid these places for a while.

5. Try to eat at the same place at the table as much as is possible. And make it comfortable for yourself.

6. Choose food which requires a knife and fork and not what you can eat with your hands. In that way it takes more time to eat. You can lower the pace at which you eat by putting your knife and fork down when chewing and only picking them up when your mouth is empty. This will make you feel like you have had enough earlier.

7. The time just after a meal is often the most difficult period. The best remedy at such a moment is to look for distractions.

8. Drink two liters of water every day. This is important because you can think that you are hungry, while you are actually thirsty. It also gives you energy and cleans your body of waste products.

9. Make a weekly menu and plan your grocery shopping. Go to the supermarket only once a week, after you have eaten. Buy fresh products, once or twice in between. Choose especially nutritious foods that are tasty and preferably sold already divided into small portions.

10. Don't keep a large stock of food in the house as long as you are still struggling with binge eating. Also, don't

plan for unexpected guests, because that "unexpected guest" always seems to be yourself.

11. Make sure you have a regular sleeping pattern. Don't do stressful things in the evening and go to bed on time. Sleep for a maximum of eight hours and take time in the morning to start the day relaxed.

12. Exercise daily for at least thirty minutes to increase energy, to get rid of your waste products and to activate the "happy hormone" endorphin. Avoid, however, exercising compulsively.

13. Plan your daily activities so that there is a balance between activity and relaxation. Avoid being bored, but also don't try to do too much. Avoid the energy gluttons as much as is possible. Put the accent on energy givers that do not go together with food (see chapter 3.)

14. Every day do at least one thing that you like and that has nothing to do with food.

15. Don't consider yourself a failure when something fails; every moment is a new chance. Emphasize the things that did go well!

16. If you let the scale decide how you feel, try to get on it less (maximum once a week on the same day and at the same time).

17. If you are overweight and you want to change your diet, remember that such a thing is meaningful only when you first have a normal eating pattern. You can start to exercise more though.

18. Postpone all important decisions until you feel better about yourself.

19. You have a self-healing ability that rises above all science, but sometimes it is very hard to get to that by yourself. Others see your blind spots better than you do. Although this frightens you, try to trust someone who will and can respectfully support you. Consider that you probably wouldn't mind listening to a loving friend talk to you about her problems.

20. When you have chronic symptoms go to your GP.

Appendix 2

Suggestions for partner and loved ones.

Supporting someone with compulsive eating behavior is not simple. Although you try to handle it as well as is possible, it is not easy. Maybe the following suggestions will help you. Realize that there is no instant recipe. Everyone is different, so every situation must be assessed separately, to determine what the right thing is to do. Further, it depends on how close you are to that person. If there is a lack of trust, then even the best suggestions can have the opposite effect.

1. Compulsive eating behavior cannot be dissolved by willpower. If it was that easy then there would not be so many people struggling with it for so long. More causes underlie it. Don't be judgmental toward her. It crept into her life and before she knew it, it started to control her life completely. Don't judge yourself either. Nobody is perfect.

2. Put the discussion about food and weight on hold. Don't try to cheer her up or minimize the eating problem by saying, "It is not that bad after all." Don't force her into a different eating pattern. This will only raise her feelings of guilt. On top of that, she would have to resort to poor

excuses and then a situation of mutual distrust will arise. Don't give unsolicited advice, like "You just have to stop binge eating."

3. Offer a listening ear; see the poem "Be Quiet" on page 221 of this book.

4. She needs unconditional support. Try to accept her as she is and show understanding and confidence. Look at her good sides.

5. Someone who demonstrates compulsive eating behavior has lost control of her life. Encouragement and warmth coming from the knowledge that you believe in her may help to point her life in a new direction.

6. She needs to feel secure. A regular daily routine and quiet surroundings are important.

7. A woman who demonstrates compulsive eating behavior is often insecure. It is possible she can't put her finger on someone else's feelings and draws wrong conclusions from them. Indicate as honestly and openly as possible what you think and feel. Accept your own feelings of sorrow, anger, fear or powerlessness and dare to talk about it.

8. Try to avoid disturbing the balance between you. That may seem impossible sometimes, but make sure that you don't act more caring than necessary. Don't take over her responsibility, because then chances are that she will lose respect for you. Support is important, but the responsibility for healing lies with her.

9. Set clear boundaries and stick to them. With this you are offering her something to rely on in her insecurity. Take care that she is not using her eating problem as an excuse

to withdraw from social obligations. Nobody profits from it when you allow her to completely control your life.

10. Don't demand too much from yourself. It is also important to take time for yourself. If you are doing well, that is also in her interest.

11. Often she is not conscious of her own needs, but is especially focused on pleasing others. Encourage her to do things that are of interest to her (and not to you).

12. It is possible that she is hesitant to try something because she is afraid of not doing it "perfectly." Try gradually to lead her away from her "black/white-world" to a world with more color nuances.

13. If she is upset because, in her eyes, she made a mistake, remind her that it is the most normal thing in the world and that, in spite of that, you still love her.

14. Try to be patient, because then you are more capable of being there for her. Acknowledge that someone with compulsive eating behavior does not intentionally want to make things difficult for you. Her behavior is caused by worrying, fears and obsessions that hardly ever are controllable. Do not take negative remarks personally, but learn to deal objectively with them.

15. Don't create feelings of guilt with comments like: "Do you understand what you are doing to me with this?" It is already difficult enough for her without all that reproach. Besides there is a strong chance that she already blames herself for what she is doing to you.

16. Don't force promises. If she can't keep to them, it will bring new feelings of guilt. Don't let you yourself be tempted to make promises that you can't keep.

17. Be an example to her when it comes to keeping things in perspective. For instance: missed the train? "That's too bad, we'll just wait quietly for the next one."

18. Don't allow her to be too hard on herself for often irrational or even rational shortcomings. Encourage her to concentrate on all her positive attributes.

19. Read about these problems.

20. Find support for yourself if necessary.

Appendix 3

The thought scheme.

Every thought that hinders you from reaching your most important goal is worth challenging.

Event + Thoughts =Feelings + Behavior

Describe briefly the event in which you had a unsatisfying and unwanted feeling. What were your expectations?

1. *Write down the automatic thoughts you had immediately after it, although you think it is good for nothing. Keep the sentences short and simple.*

2. *Challenge*

   - Is this really true? What are the arguments in favor of those automatic thoughts?

   - What are the arguments against those automatic thoughts?

   - Is it in my interest to think like that? Yes/no, because

   - Is it good for my health? (psychological/physical) Yes/ no, because

- What is my most important goal?

- Will I reach my goal with these automatic thoughts? Yes/no, because

- What can I do to reach my goal?

- How will I feel when I have reached my goal?

3. *My newest realistic thought is:*

Appendix 4

Goal.

Goal:

Step 1: in the period from . . . until . . . I will do the following:

    Evaluation: Did I carry out the step as I planned it?

    Did I reach my goal with it?

Step 2: In the period from . . . until . . . I will do the following:

    Evaluation: Did I carry out the step as I planned it?

    Did I reach my goal with it?

Step 3: In the period from . . . until . . . I will do the following:

    Evaluation: Did I carry out the step as I planned it?

    Did I reach my goal with it?

Appendix 5

What do I really hunger for?

When we have no physical hunger we can first ask ourselves with every difficult moment what the reason is that we want to eat. We can do that with the help of the next questions:

1. In what situation am I? (Try to observe the situation as purely as possible, without interpretation, comparison or labeling).

2. Which thoughts do I have? Challenge immediately irrational thoughts! (See also "Realistic thinking" in chapter 2.)

3. What do I feel?

4. What is my real need?

5. How can I fulfill that need?

6. How will I feel then?

7. What will be changed in a positive way over a year if I take my life in my own hands now?

Notes

Chapter 1

1. Scientifically mapped by psychologist and researcher Elaine Aron. The title of her first book is *The Highly Sensitive Person* (Carol Publishing Group, Secaucus).

2. This is also the experience of my colleagues Peggy-Claude Pierre, *The Secret Language of Eating Disorders* (Times Books, New York) and Anita Johnston, *Eating in the Light of the Moon* (Birch Lane Press, Secaucus).

Chapter 2

3. These nine basic patterns are based on the philosophy of the wise Armenian teacher, G.I. Gurdjieff (1865–1949), who was inspired by Sufism and sources going back to Babylon circa 2500 B.C. It is not my intention to present a complete picture of "the limited self." It is only meant to provide an insight into the manifold aspects of our personalities, which most clients will recognize.

4. Marginal note for family, friends and social workers: often, in the beginning, the psychological condition of the client militates against asking for help. As a result, it makes the client a victim. One should not think in a negative way; positive perceptions should be strengthened. Foolish demands of oneself work against oneself, whereas positive notions encourage patience and love.

Chapter 4

5. Sometimes, allowing yourself to eat can make you so tense that it is important for you to divert your thoughts and not focus on the source of your tension.

6. The first thing to remember is to feel what your needs are at this very moment. Only after that can you bid farewell to all illusions, to old or unfulfilled "child longings" and let them be what they are, namely unattainable.

7. In modern medical terminology, extreme forms of "pica" are defined under DSM-IV-TR-307. 52, meaning a psychiatric aberration. In practice, a milder tendency to "strange urges" was also characterized as "pica," which is the Latin word for a magpie, a bird which is omnivorous.

Chapter 6

8. It would require a much larger book than this one to go more deeply into this matter. However, In the literature section, you will find listed a book on this family therapy.

Chapter 7

9. The quotation by Pantanjali is from *Crises and the Miracle of Love* by Mansukh Patel and Helena Waters (Life Foundation Publications, Bilston, England).

10. While we dream, research has shown, the part of the brain that deals with social adjustments is hardly activated. In our dreams, this part of the will is practically always switched off.

Literature

Elaine Aron, *The Highly Sensitive Person* (Carol Publishing Group, Secaucus).

Peggy Claude-Pierre, *The Secret Language of Eating Disorders* (Times Books, New York).

Bert Hellinger, *Love's Hidden Symmetry* (Zeig Tucker & Theisen Publishers).

Anita Johnston, *Eating in the Light of the Moon* (Birch Lane Press, Secaucus).

Mansukh Patel and Helena Waters, *Crisis and the Miracle of Love* (Life Foundation Publications, Bilston, England).

Clarissa Pinkola Estés, *Women Who Run with the Wolves* (Ballantine, New York).

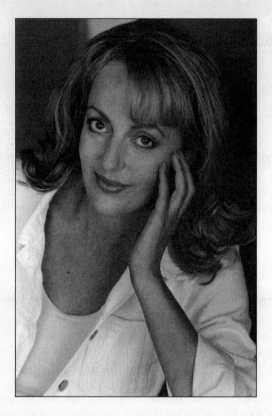

For more information about Joanna Kortink's
work see www.joannakortink.com